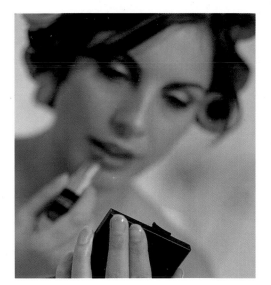

superflirt

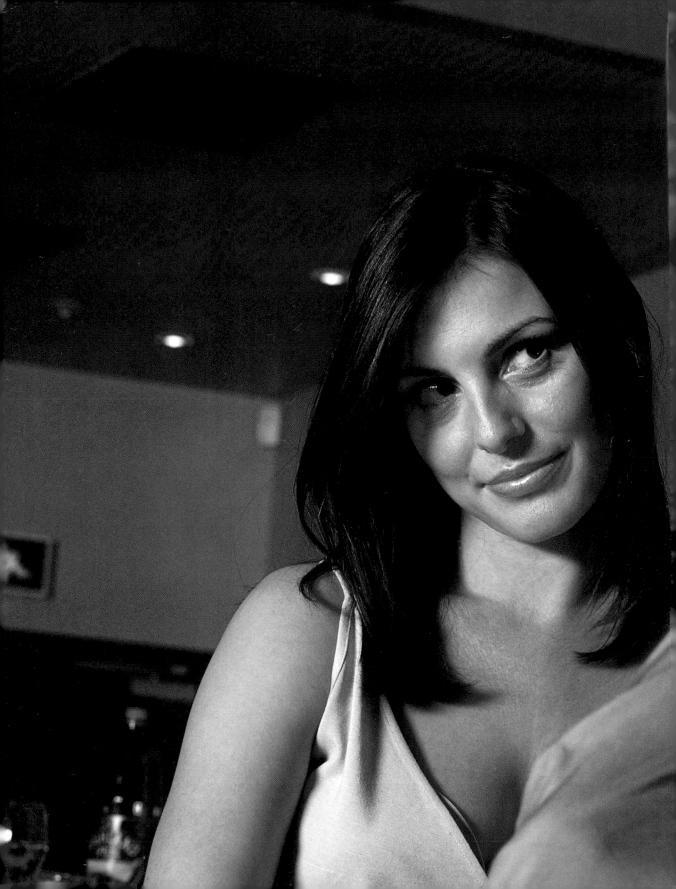

superflirt
tracey cox

photography by
janeanne gilchrist at unit photographic

DK Publishing

LONDON, NEW YORK, MUNICH, MELBOURNE, DELHI

Design
KAB Design
Senior Editor
Peter Jones
Managing Art Editor
Emma Forge
Category Publisher
Corinne Roberts
Art Director
Carole Ash
DTP Designer
Karen Constanti
Production Controller
Heather Hughes
Production Manager
Lauren Britton
Jacket Editor
Beth Apple
Jacket Designer
Katy Wall

For my mentor, Desmond Morris, the
master of nonverbal communication

First American Edition, 2003
Published in the United States by
DK Publishing, Inc.
375 Hudson Street
New York, New York 10014

03 04 05 06 07 08 10 9 8 7 6 5 4 3 2 1

Library of Congress
Cataloging in Publication Division
101 Independence Ave., S.E.
Washington, D.C. 20540-4320
Library of Congress Cataloging-in-Publication
Data

Cox, Tracey.
Superflirt / Tracey Cox ;
photography by Unit 21.
p. cm.
            Includes index.
            ISBN 0-7894-9651-8 (alk. paper)
            1.Man-woman relationships. 2.
Interpersonal attraction. 3. Body Language. 4.
Nonverbal communication. I. Title.

    HQ801.C7382003
    306.7 --dc21

2003051672

ISBN 0-7894-9651-8

Color reproduction by GRB, Italy
Printed and bound in Gütersloh, Germany
by MOHNMEDIA, GmbH

Discover more at
www.dk.com

contents

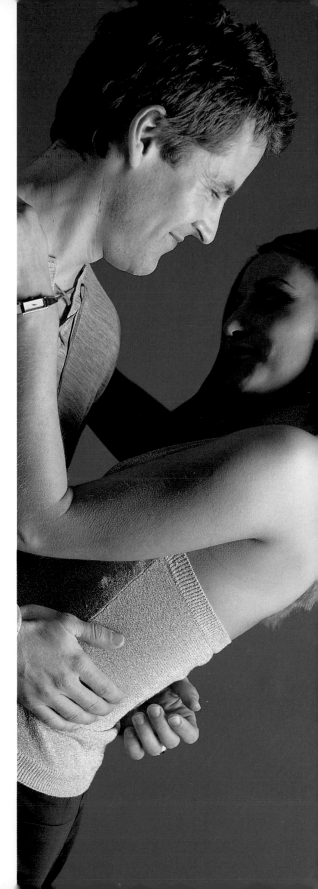

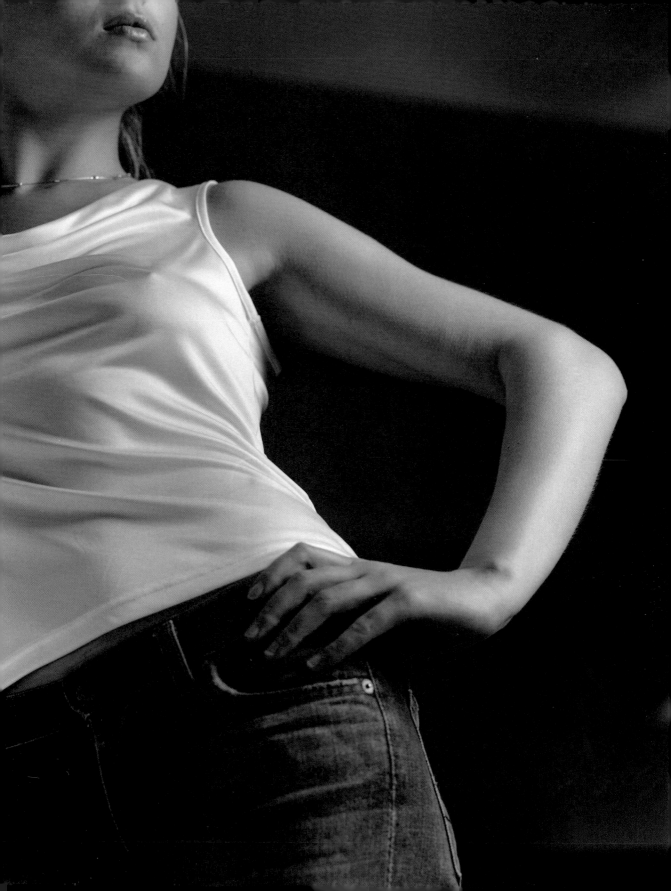

Introduction

Flirting gets a lot of bad press. "It's degrading!" sniff some. "Surely we've progressed beyond the batting eyelashes stuff." "It's about playing games and I hate games," say others. "If they don't like me as I am, that's their problem." And then the old classic…"Flirting's for bimbos and himbos. It's unintelligent." Oh, puhleeze! Flirting isn't any of the above—it's just damn good fun for everyone involved.

I admit it: I'm a shameless flirt. I flirt with men, women, dogs, cats, babies, and ladybugs. I'd flirt with a lamppost if no one else stood still for long enough. Flirting's fun—that's why people do it. It isn't about playing games. It's not really even about picking someone up (although it's a damn good way to do it). Today's flirt is simply yesterday's charmer renamed. Superflirts aren't sleazy, cheesy, or intrusive. They just let others know they find them interesting. They're playful, adventurous, open, friendly, warm, lovable, sizzlingly sexy, and, above all, popular. What's not to like? A good flirt makes people feel good.

> I admit it: **I'm a shameless flirt**…I'd flirt with a lamppost if no one else **stood still for long** enough

Master the techniques in *superflirt* and it could dramatically alter your love life and all your relationships. The book's primarily aimed at romantic liaisons, but the skills covered can enhance your relationships with everyone. I'm going to show you techniques to make you irresistible to the opposite sex (or the same sex, if you prefer). I'll teach you how to let someone know you're attracted to them without saying a word—and how to tell if the feeling's mutual. The idea is to make you more likeable and attractive to everyone by teaching you how to interpret your own body language (so you're sending the signals you want) and decode other people's (to learn their true feelings).

That's the good news. Now brace yourself, because change is hard. If your body language and flirting skills need readjustment, teaching your body different ways to stand, sit, and walk often feels contrived and unnatural at the start. This is entirely normal. After all, your body has been used to behaving in a certain way your entire life! Happily, it takes just six weeks to retrain your body and rid yourself of old habits. That's six weeks to become a superflirt. Worth a try, don't you think?

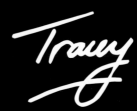

1

BODY BASICS

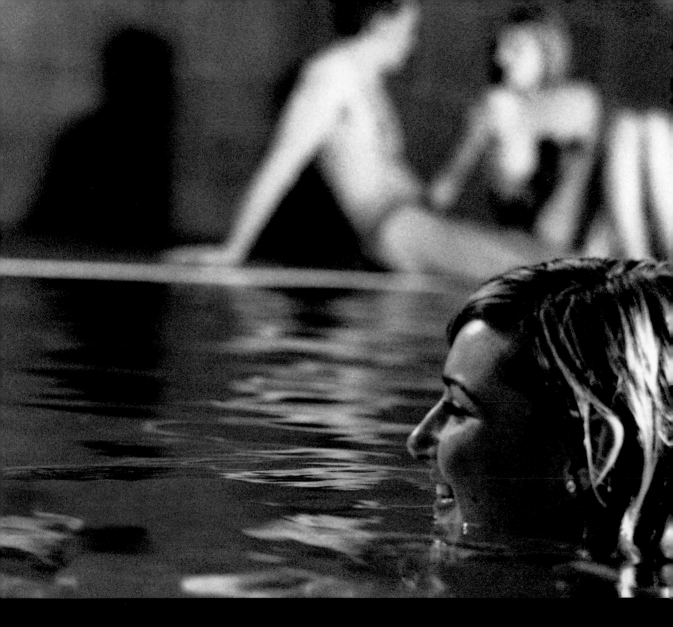

Get what you want without saying a word. Plus tips on how to talk to strangers, **invade someone's space,** eye up the talent, **and turn someone on**—in a mere 10 seconds

Fake it till you make it

Get what you want without saying a word

Alter your body language to look and feel instantly sexier and more confident. Learn how to interpret *other's* gestures and you could find out if they're attracted to you, before they even know it themselves.

Stop someone on the street and ask them how humans communicate and it's likely they'll answer, "With words." The truth is, we signal around 12 things silently for every message delivered verbally. Almost all researchers agree that 65 percent of communication is through nonverbal body language— lots claim it's more like 90 percent! Some of these body language signals we're conscious of making— giving a friend the thumbs up after they've made a great speech or winking at someone to share a private joke. Most, we're not. We all subconsciously send out a constant stream of other gestures that reveal our innermost thoughts and feelings. The way we walk, stand, sit, and hold ourselves reflects our perspective on life and how it's treated us. First impressions are hard to shake because they're often accurate—our body language reflects our personality in ways most of us aren't even aware of!

If you find all that a little alarming, join the club. When I was first presented with this evidence, I too wanted to sit on my hands and not move a muscle ever again. Especially not in front of anyone I was remotely attracted to. Did this mean the guy sitting next to me at work could read my mind? Were my secret fantasies written all over my face? The answer is "yes." If he knew enough about body language, he probably would be able to read the secret signals that give away lust and infatuation, effectively seeing through the ultra-cool façade to spot the true emotions (lust) jostling just below the surface. Yikes! How embarrassing is that? Then something else occurred to me: if he can learn to "read" what I'm really thinking, then I must be able to read him. And for anyone who's ever thought, "I wonder what they think about me?" this is damn handy.

There's even more good news. Reading body language isn't just priceless when you're looking for a pickup, interpreting your own body language can help you recognize hidden emotions bubbling just below the surface. It also makes you aware of what signals you're sending others, helping you understand their reactions to you. Positively adjusting or actively altering your body language when you're dealing with others can drastically up your chances of them liking, loving, or respecting you, often allowing you to get what you want without saying a word! How? Understanding body language allows you to gather information about people's feelings which they're too shy, polite, or uptight to admit, or aren't even aware of themselves. An eyebrow flash (see p.86) lets you know someone's interested before they've even registered the thought themselves. Care for a flingette?

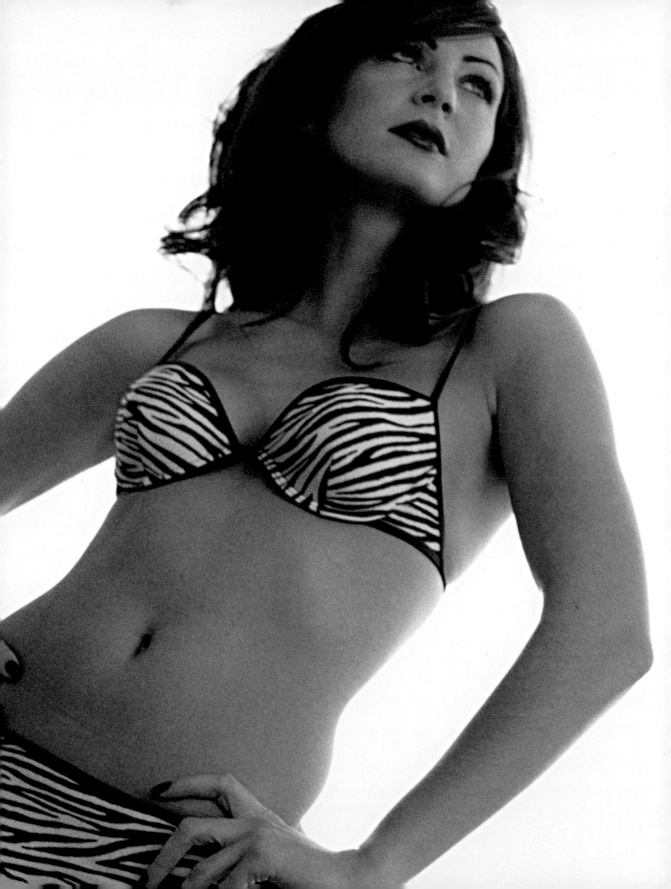

Want a long-term partner? Want to make yourself generally more popular, confident, and authoritative? I can't think of a more effective way to do it than to master the art of body language.

A lot of what I'm going to talk about in this book relies on the "fake it till you make it" principle. This simply means that if you alter your body language, you can alter your attitude, perceptions, and emotions. Yes, I know you're thinking "Can't she just fast-forward to the eyebrow flash part and skip the theory?" and I promise to do just that in a nanosecond. But there are a few basics you need to understand if you're going to be really, really good at it, and this is one of them. Because our body language reflects our personality, it follows that particular gestures and behaviors are

Change your **body language** and the mind often follows. **Walk tall** and your **self-esteem lifts** as well.

associated with particular personalities. The simplest example of all is this: happy people smile, angry people frown. Put a smile on your face and people will assume you're happy; frown and they'll assume you're not. If you therefore imitate or adopt the body language gestures of the personality you'd like to have, you'll be seen as having that personality. Let's say you're shy. Act confident: stand up straight and look people in the eye, and people will think you're confident because that's how confident people behave. Now here's the magical part: because you're acting confident, people will now think you are. Never mind that inside you're a complete mess—all they see is a cool, confident exterior. This affects the way they react to you. Confident people get asked for their opinions, so it's likely you will be too. And while you may be a bit nervous and surprised because this doesn't normally happen, you'll probably manage to volunteer something and—"Wow! I did it!"—suddenly, you feel just a little bit important. You start to feel confident and so the chain reaction continues. Initially you're faking it—pretending with your body language to be something you're not. Do it long enough, however, and eventually your body language will reflect the real you because you've become that person. Get it? I hope so!

Don't get me wrong, I'm all for working on the cause not the symptom: you need to address the issues that made you shy in the first place, as well as work on your body language. But whoever said there was an order to how we should improve ourselves? We think too much sometimes. So how about you bypass the brain for a bit, forget about what you feel like on the inside, and instead work on an outward illusion? Personally, I think it's more sensible. Change your body language and the mind often follows. Walk tall and your self-esteem lifts as well. Facial expressions are equally as mood-altering. It's called "the facial feedback effect": our expressions reinforce the emotion that caused them because the position of our facial muscles feeds information back to our brain. Stretch your mouth into a smile and the brain registers that we're smiling and releases the hormonal response that usually accompanies a real smile and feeling happy. Our "happy face" and "feeling happy" works backward as well as forward.

Hopefully, this goes some way toward answering those who think it's being "false" to use body language or anything else that improves our external appearance because "it's what's inside that counts" and "it's bad or manipulative to pretend to be something you're not." Listen, I'm all for letting it all hang out once people get to know each other, but I vehemently believe, for certain situations such as dates, job interviews, and meeting the parents, that it's in everyone's interest to present themselves in the best possible light. Most people make an effort to look good and be on their best behavior in those circumstances—particularly on a date. And with good reason. What's underneath is important, but you've got to look OK and get the body language right for your date to want to stick around and see what else you've got to offer.

There's something else that tends to get brought up when body language is mentioned. There's always someone who says, "It's all just garbage. I crossed my arms just then and it was because I was cold, not defensive. See, I tricked you!" Not. Anyone who tries to read someone based on

> ## What's **underneath is important**, but you've got to look OK for a date to want to stick around and see **what else you've got to offer.**

one body language gesture, is barking mad. Everyone has their own personalized body language— the reason why the Rule of Four is so important (see p.150). The idea is to look for clusters of gestures—lots of things pointing toward the same conclusion—rather than just one thing. It's not an infallible science, and it certainly won't tell you everything—we need words as well. But it is an astonishingly subtle and effective way to gather information. It could even help you predict the future of your relationship! Psychologist and relationships guru John Gottman studied 700 married couples over a long period. Part of his research involved videotaping the couples discussing stressful issues in their relationship or reminiscing about how they met. Afterward, he analyzed their body language, focusing on facial expressions (including real vs. fake smiles, curled upper lips, and rolling eyes). Based on what he learned from this, Gottman is now able to predict with 75 percent accuracy, whether a couple will divorce within six years, simply by analyzing three minutes of body language interaction on video. Give him 15 minutes and his accuracy score climbs to 85 percent. Now that's impressive!

Walking the **walk...**

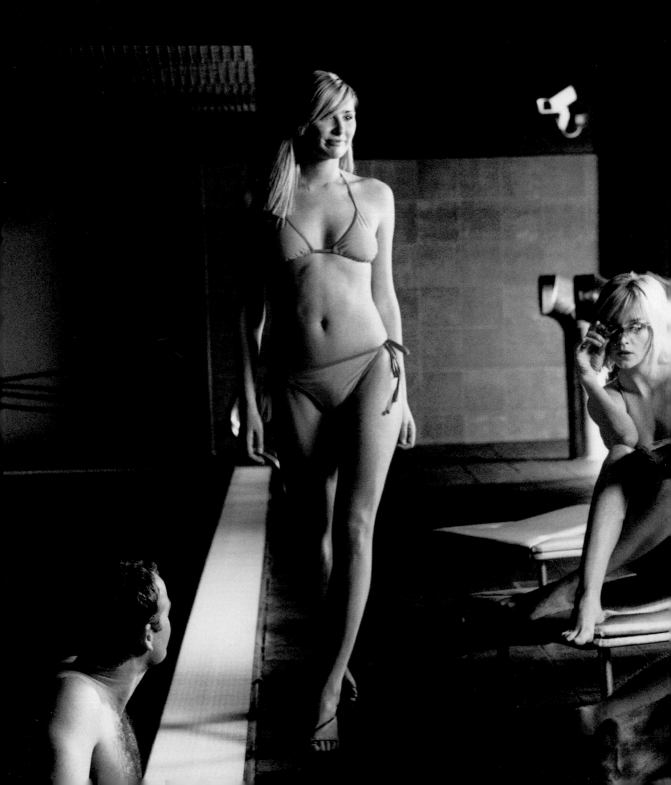

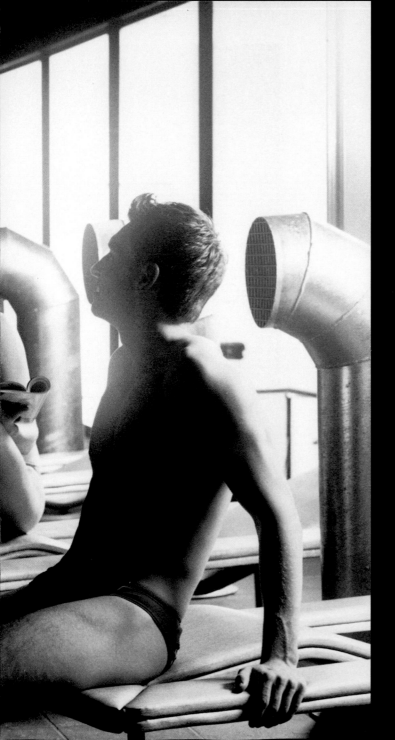

Aside from boasting a spectacular body, the girl in the orange bikini has got a walk to match. The exaggerated roll of her hips, the squared shoulders, saucily swinging arms, direct eye contact, and ultra-confident facial expression all work together to produce dramatic results. If our body language reflects the way we feel about ourselves, this girl's having a great hair day! The higher our self-esteem, the higher we hold ourselves (actual height doesn't matter—it's presence and attitude that count). The way we walk is such an accurate indicator of personality and mood, that mirroring someone's walk is one of the quickest ways to glean clues about their true character. By imitating and getting "in step" with another person for mere minutes, you can understand their world and get a taste of what it feels like to be them. Walk in a stressed person's shoes—fast, with purpose, looking straight ahead, and rarely distracted—and you'll also start to feel anxious. Mirror an ambler, who doesn't just smell the roses but stops to plant a few, and the anxiety dissolves into a hazy whatever-whenever horizon. If you're like most people, this information will both intrigue and terrify you. On the one hand, it's handy to know if you're desperately trying to bond with someone new. On the other, it's alarming. If your walk is a giveaway, what messages are you sending each time you put one foot in front of the other? Turn to find out.

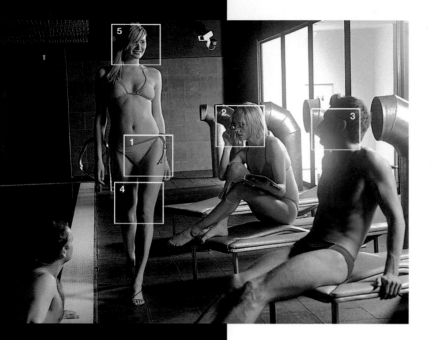

Are you putting

What comes first?

We all lead with a part of our body when we walk—it's the bit that looks as though it's being pulled forward, ahead of everything else. Lead with your shoulders and you'll look protective and fearful. Lead with your knees and your legs look like they're carrying you places you don't want to go. If your chest enters the room before you do, you're at a risk of appearing pushy. The two best options for maximum effectiveness? A neutral walk—where no body part leads—or to lead with your pelvis.

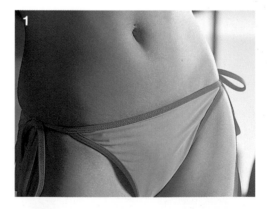

Rolling hips (1) A hip-swinging walk sends a powerful me-Jane, you-Tarzan sexual signal. Anatomical differences mean women have a greater rolling action of the pelvis. Switched-on females know rolling hips draw attention to hips, butt, and genitals, and can mean the difference between attracting attention or being ignored.

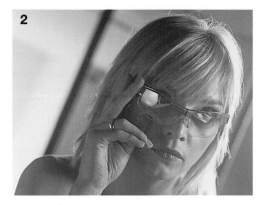

The jealous checkout (2) Though equally as good-looking, the seated blonde is aware she's been thoroughly upstaged. Her legs give away her true feelings through intention movements. One leg draws protectively toward her body to self-comfort; the other steps out toward her rival, wanting to literally follow in her footsteps.

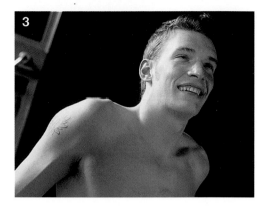

Undisguised admiration (3) With arms spread wide open, this man's assumed the classic "seduce me" position. Confronted with a gorgeous, sexually aggressive woman, his head tilts upward ready to be kissed, and his body leans slightly backward as a clear invitation for her to pounce and have her wicked way.

your best foot forward?

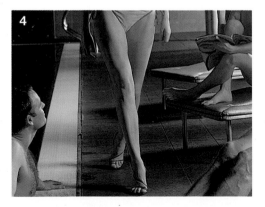

Long legs (4) Our legs account for roughly half our body's height, aptly illustrated if you mentally locate the central point—the tie of this girl's bikini bottoms on her thigh. An exposed length of leg is sexy for one simple reason— the more you see, the more likely you are to imagine the point where they meet.

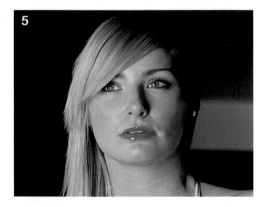

Head held high (5) A confident, raised head is a typical high-status display of a dominant individual. Check out the main photo and you'll also see her shoulders are thrust back, her pelvis is thrust forward, and she's forcing others to look up to her when meeting her gaze.

The 10-second turn-on

Within 10 seconds, the person you're meeting will have made up their mind about what sort of person they think you are. Scared? You should be. This first impression is based entirely on what you look like and how you move and hold yourself. Ten seconds. This means before they've even had time to process a rational thought, they've made up their mind about you. (Studies show we feel emotional reactions before the brain has time to register what's caused them.) If this doesn't send you running to the nearest mirror for a quick body check, it should. Even the "it's what's inside that counts" lobby has to agree—it's worth doing an external once-over because our body language reflects our personalities.

Every movement we make **exposes our private thoughts,** who we are, what we're thinking, our dreams, **ambitions, and fears. Gulp.**

It's impossible not to communicate. Even when you say nothing, you say something. Posture and body language tell the story of our life: whether we've been happy or sad, a survivor or a victim. Every movement we make exposes our past and our current private thoughts: who we are, what we're thinking, our dreams, ambitions, and fears. Gulp. Now, if simply standing in front of someone means you're effectively handing over your autobiography, it makes sense to check that your body is doing a good job of it. Get into the habit of running through a mental posture checklist, and the next time the stopwatch starts ticking, you'll be confident your body's presenting you in the best possible light.

STAND UP FOR YOURSELF
It's quite difficult to get a true picture of how you really stand and walk because the minute that we see a mirror, all of us tend to straighten up. We pull our tummies in, our shoulders go back, and we assume the facial expression that we think is our most flattering. To get a truer picture, try walking toward a full-length mirror with your eyes averted, then stand in front of it with your eyes shut. Picture yourself at a party with friends, get into position, and then open your eyes and take a look. Ask friends to be honest about their impression of the way that you stand, sit, and walk and when you're in important situations, every 10 minutes or so, get into the habit of looking down to see what your body is doing. The following are some of the things that you should be aware of:

THE PERSONALITY AND PAST CHECK
Not great One glance and it will be pretty obvious what kind of life you've had. If it's been a hard road, you'll invariably have rounded, slumped shoulders (they collapse under the weight of excessive responsibility). People who've gone through prolonged periods of depression still stoop

and sag years after they've recovered. The lines on our faces also tell a story: if you've spent much of your life worried or frowning,, the results are etched on your forehead and the corners of your mouth turn down. Shy, scared people fold in on themselves. Their shoulders try to meet across their chest, arms fold across their body—in effect, they're trying to make themselves look as small as possible. Clenched fists, a tight jaw, rigid spine, and shoulders lifted so high, they're practically around your ears are all trademarks of a tense, highly anxious person.

Better While it's impossible to alter the past, the present is very much in your control. Alter nothing else but your attitude toward your life and you'll still notice an extraordinary difference. Do you want people to see you as more confident—a force to be reckoned with? Do what dominant people do: draw yourself up to look as big, tall, and noticeable as possible! Want to appear as a winner rather than victim? Again, hold your head high, put your shoulders back, and meet your own eyes in the mirror. Now, keep the same position, but take a deep breath and let your body relax into it. Uncross everything. Smile. Fantastic!

THE MOOD CHECK

Not great Your posture reflects your mood quite literally: if you're feeling down, everything slumps and droops. If you're submissive, your head hangs and you'll avoid meeting people's eyes. Also watch how your body faces the people you're talking to: if you're not sure you're really welcome, you'll tend to stand with your body turned side-on, rather than square-on.

Better If you're feeling up and happy, you really do have a spring in your step, stand tall, and try to reach the sky. When we're relaxed, our legs and arms aren't symmetrical—we'll lean one arm on the back of a chair or prop ourselves up. We also tend to lean sideways and slightly backward, shifting our weight so it's distributed comfortably.

THE BODY IMAGE CHECK

Not great Compare the postures of teenage girls and you'll see plenty of examples of this one. The girl who's ashamed of developing breasts will hunch forward, fold her arms, and let her (usually long) hair fall as a curtain to hide both her face and the offending items. A few years on, when she's figured breasts are A Good Thing, she'll do the opposite: throw her head back, push her chest forward, and remove her arms so that people can admire them. Everyone has yuk-I-hate-my-body days—and it's always obvious. If you're not hugging a pillow or bag to your chest in an effort to hide your stomach, you're looking acutely uncomfortable by pulling at too-tight clothing or trying not to look swamped by clothing which is too big. All of which accomplishes the opposite to what's intended: people's eyes are drawn to what's causing all the activity or acute embarrassment.

Better If you've got serious body image issues, try to get some counseling (at least read the do-it-yourself sex makeover, pp.64–69). Or take refuge in the "spotlight" theory—that people are far too busy worrying about their own appearance to even notice yours! Put on an outfit that you feel comfortable in, avoid fiddling and hiding the supposed problem areas, and I guarantee that no one will notice a single flaw!

Gender menders

Why our body parts affect the way we flirt

Quite frankly, I don't buy the whole men-are-from-Mars, women-are-from-Venus thing. But there are differences we can't escape—and not just the obvious (like genitals). Anatomy, the way we're brought up, which side of the brain we use—all are genuine differences. Happily though, it really is a case of *vive la différence*! All can be solved with a little understanding and readjustment.

I remember, quite soon into a relationship, this guy I was dating showed up early at my house.—I was still getting ready and it felt mean to leave him in the living room on his own, so I said "Come and talk to me while I put my makeup on." He dutifully followed me into the bathroom, then after about two seconds blurted out "Would you mind if I watched TV?" "Fine," I said, but rather huffily. I took that as a complete lack of interest. He'd rather watch football than talk to me, and obviously wasn't interested in moving things on to a more intimate level. After all, there's something distinctly long-termish about chatting with a man while layering on the mascara. Turned out I was wrong on all counts. "Things like that terrify blokes," he confessed later. "I don't know how to talk to you while you're putting on makeup. Where do I look? At you or in the mirror? Where would I sit? Should I say I got turned on when you were putting on lipstick? I knew I'd screw it up somehow, so I just got out of there." As someone who regularly gets up on the soapbox to argue how similar the sexes are rather than "alien," it was a bit of a wake-up call. While (to me anyway) it's still glaringly obvious that men and women are mostly alike once you remove their genitals (figuratively speaking, of course), we sometimes look at the world through different eyes.

"That's the understatement of the millennium," grumbles my friend John, victim of a recent date debacle. "I'm out with a girl who's got on a top which is so low, I can see where her nipples start! Call me shallow, but I'm slightly distracted by this and end up asking her the same question several times over. She was so insulted, believing that I wasn't listening to her, that we end up having a fight. So why did she wear that top then, if she didn't want me to look?," he said mystified. I mumbled something about fashion but in the end had to agree with him. I've gone out with friends sporting spectacular cleavage and when face-to-face with a pair of half-exposed breasts, jiggling and jumping around and taking on a life of their own with every movement, I can't help but stare, too. (Moral of story: if you've got something important to say to him, do it in a polo-neck.)

It's partly the differences in the male and female body shape—breasts attached to our chests, a penis swinging from his groin— that explains why the sexes tend to use different body language

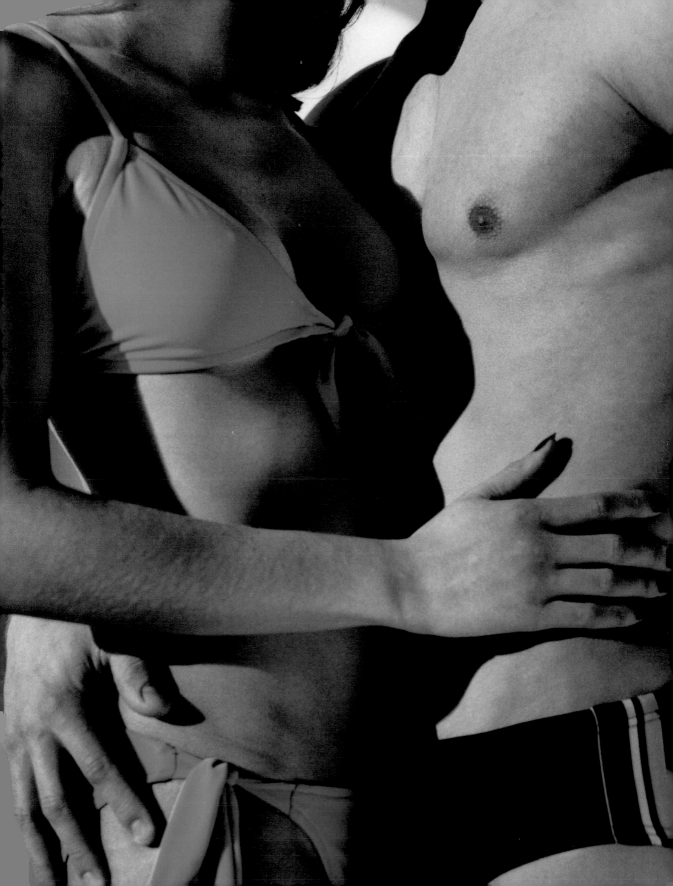

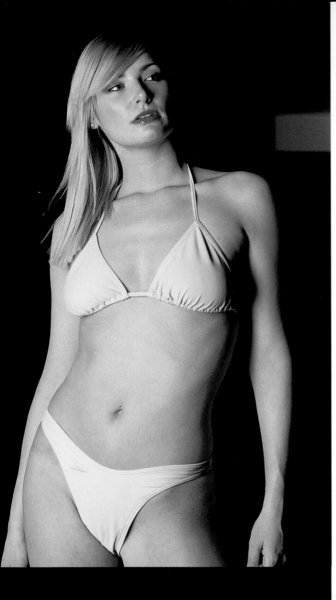

The average female will send out five times **more sexual signals** than the average man.

and flirting signals. Her fingers, seductively stroking her neck then trailing down toward her cleavage, gets men fired up because her hand's on its way to her breasts. His big, beefy hand fighting its way through a tangle of chest hair, doesn't quite have the same effect. Ditto things like crossing and uncrossing your legs. Women often sit with one leg wrapped around the other. You try doing a leg twine with two testicles in the way! Genitals apart, men are generally taller, heavier, and bigger than women simply because….they're men. After all, our bodies are built for function and men are the original hunters. They needed longer and larger feet so they could run faster, broader shoulders and longer arms to balance and aim weapons, stronger skulls and thicker jaws to protect them against predators. Women also needed certain physical attributes to keep up their end of the deal (to populate the earth in return for food, protection, and the odd nut and berry). In retrospect, I'm not sure this was a fair swap. Given the choice, I think I'd have gone for the odd scuffle with a wild beast versus periods, pregnancy, and childbirth. Anyway, the reason why women have wide pelvises and breasts, smaller waists, thicker thighs, and a longer belly is that these features all assist in childbearing. Because there was no need for them to appear big and scary to potential attackers, women take up less space than men and keep their limbs closer to their bodies. They have narrow shoulders and smaller upper arms. A man's arms often appear to dangle in space, held away from his body by the bulk of muscle in his upper arm…well, they do if he's been a good boy and gone to the gym.

These evolutionary physical differences can make a mockery of unisex. The modern male might not be out hunting prey, the modern woman might not be stuck at home as a breeding machine, but our bodies still behave as if they were. It's hard to stop doing something when you're not aware you're doing it, and our body shape and size still dictate our movements. Besides, men still chase symbolic prey in business and women still satisfy deep maternal urges. "Change they will," writes Desmond Morris sagely, "but it'll take another million years of evolution to become a genetic reality."

Recent research based on people moving through crowds highlights other body language differences in genders. Hidden cameras show women usually turn away from men as they push past, men turn toward females. She's protecting her breasts and (this is my take on it), he's hoping for a quick brush against them. Women spend more time touching their hair than men do and are more likely to clasp their hands. Men are more likely to fold their arms across their chests and hug via a shoulder embrace; women opt for fuller contact body hugs. Other gender differences we previously thought were learned, but it looks like they might well be innate. UK researchers recently reported the results of long-term studies on 3,000 sets of twins. As early as two years old, girls outperformed boys on cognitive scores—especially verbal ability— and remained consistently superior in a wide range of verbal tasks. To outperform at such a young age appears to put paid to the theory that women end up more articulate through learned behavior (i.e., parents talk more to girls than boys).

Then there's sex. Long before we're remotely interested in what our sexual organs are for, and light-years away from the point when we decide to use them for procreation rather than recreation, we're given gender identities by society and by our parents. Equal opportunity, yeah right…girls and

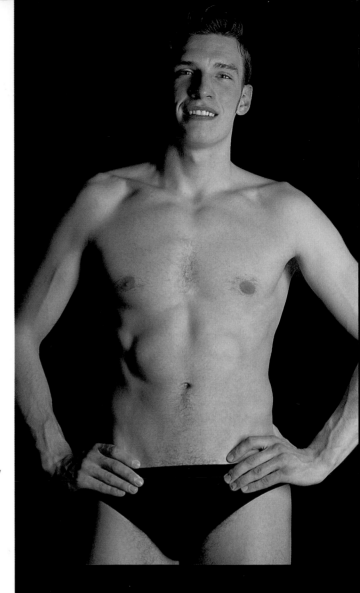

Men use **teasing and sarcasm** to show affection, are more argumentative, and hold fewer **grudges.**

boys are given different clothes, hairstyles, toys, sports, and hobbies from the word go. Even our attitudes toward sex can be traced back to biology. Boys begin masturbating at quite an early age—probably because their genitals are more obvious and accessible and, well, pretty difficult to ignore, really. Nearly all men can orgasm by age 15, and arousal tends to be almost exclusively focused on the penis.

Vaginas and clitorises aren't in view. In fact, unless you take a mirror and have a good look, you could go a whole lifetime without ever knowing what yours looked like. Combine this with society's view on masturbation (dirty, desperate) and sex in general (good girls don't do it too early), and plenty of women sail right through to their twenties without ever having masturbated or having an orgasm at all. (Sadly, plenty more continue to journey through life this way as well). Even those who do discover the joys of solo sex end up less genitally focused than men. Women discover that the sexy parts of us that we can see—like breasts—feel pleasurable when touched. And because girls touch more, they also learn early on how nice it feels to have their skin stroked in all kinds of places. All of which adds up to a more well-rounded sexual awareness, rather than one centered on obvious erogenous zones. Another added spin-off: women are usually more aware of the subtle sexual potential in each and every part of their body, so use all of it to send

Different body parts mean **different flirting signals.** You try doing a leg twine with **two testicles in the way.**

sexual signals, giving themselves many more at their disposal. The average female will send out five times more sexual signals than the average man! This means that a woman is often better at flirting and able to reduce a grown man to his knees with one well-timed lick of her lips. Now, what was all that about being the weaker sex?

HIS AND HERS
Men... have a larger, longer, and wider nose, and coarser skin. Testosterone makes pores expand and hairs sprout—the reason why men will spend nearly 60 days and nights of their lives shaving (that's around five minutes a day from age 15). They also interrupt more, mumble more, talk slower, offer minimal responses, use less emotional verbs, make direct accusations, favor the left side (factual, objective) of their brain, speak around 12,000 words a day, take up more space, gesture away from their body, gesture with fingers together, lean backward when listening, assume more relaxed sitting positions, make less direct eye contact, frown and squint more, open their mouths less when talking, use teasing and sarcasm to show affection, are more argumentative, hold fewer grudges, stick to the point when arguing, and are less likely to ask for help.

Women… have lighter skin, smaller heads (two-thirds the size of a man's), fuller lips, more fat on their cheeks, more prominent eyes (their eyeballs are the same size but higher, and plucked brows make the eyes look larger), confront problems more often (albeit indirectly and politely), favor the right side (feeling, intuition) of their brain, speak twice as much as men (25,000 words a day), take up less physical space, gesture toward their body, gesture with fingers apart, lean forward when listening, make more eye contact, smile and nod more when listening, open mouths more when speaking, interrupt less, are more articulate, show more affection, are less argumentative, are more likely to hold a grudge, bring up things from the past in current arguments, talk faster, use more support words and gestures, seek approval by adding tag questions (such as "isn't it?") on the end of statements, are more self critical, and apt to blame themselves.

Boys begin masturbating at quite an early age—probably because their **genitals are more accessible** and, well, pretty difficult to ignore, really. **Nearly all men can orgasm** by age 15.

Connect better with him by:
- Lowering your voice
- Being clear about what you want
- Presenting facts as a basis for an argument, not just feelings
- Not talking so fast
- Varying the subject matter—talking about things he's interested in, not just what you're into
- Making direct statements—"We need to…," not "I hope we…"
- Not apologizing just to be polite
- Not bearing grudges

Connect better with her by:
- Talking about your emotions, not just facts
- Asking her opinion
- Active listening—more "uh-huhs" and nods
- Using the dreaded "feel" word ("How do you feel about that?")
- Sitting upright and leaning forward
- Making more eye contact
- Showing more emotion
- Using more adjectives

Get noticed!

Mounting a full-frontal attack

Don't just make heads turn when you walk into a room, have them do a 360-degree swivel. Here are tips on how to really make an entrance and make yourself the person in the room everyone wants to meet.

I have to confess upfront that making an entrance is something with which I've had spectacular success. Except perhaps not in the right way. Being the world's clumsiest person, I've tripped, skidded, slid, and stumbled my way into a room so often I've ceased to be embarrassed about it. The pinnacle of humiliation though, had to be during the making of a talk show I did for Sky TV in the UK. To kick off each program, filmed live in front of an audience, I was supposed to bound energetically down a winding staircase, all the while beaming at the camera. Not realizing I fall over even while intently concentrating on where I'm going, the producers also didn't factor in another issue: I've got whopping big feet. This staircase was built for elegant little feet attached to an elegant little person, who'd come prettily trotting down with a few click-clacks of her delicate stilettos. Not Mrs. Bean on feet big enough to ski on. I tried to explain all this but they still sent me up there. So there I was, right at the top, terrified. The audience started clapping and the show music started playing and I'm thinking "How the hell can I bound when I'll be hard pressed to walk down while clinging on to the rail?" and someone's in my ear saying "10 seconds, 9 seconds…" and I have to do something, so I come stomping down, as light on my feet as an elephant, and I'm so relieved to get near the bottom without falling over that I do bound the last little bit…and that's when my feet get all wound up with the camera cords and the next minute I'm flat on my back saying a rather naughty word rather loudly. Like, "Hello, I'm the star of the show! An authoritative expert here to fix all of your problems! Take me seriously!" Not.

You'll be relieved to hear I've become a lot better at making entrances since then (And you're taking advice from this woman?), mainly due to slowing the whole thing down and following some basic principles. Barging/falling into a room, Tracey-style, won't get you very far, but then again, neither will slinking in and clinging to the corners. Enter a room that way and people will instantly brand you as someone not worth talking to. Instead, get noticed by dividing your entrance into three separate steps. (This works if you're entering solo or with friends.)

Step one Pause in the doorway with your head held high and shoulders back (if you are with friends, let them go ahead). Lazily scan the room, giving the impression that you're looking for someone. Even if you're not pretending and you spot them immediately, hover for a few seconds.

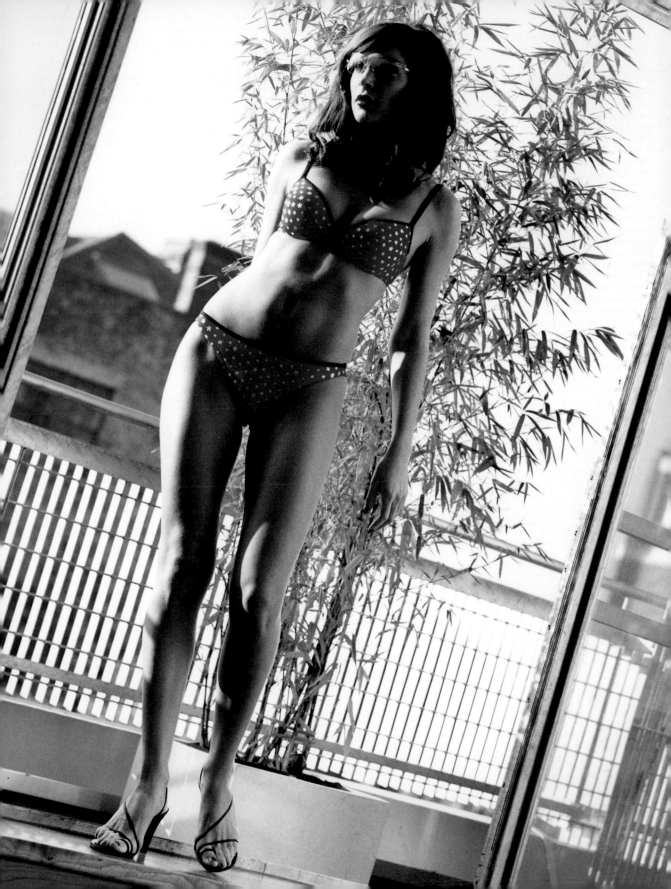

The idea is to let all potential dates/new friends/playmates get a good look at you looking your best. (Let's face it, we all sag as the night goes on!)

Step two Make eye contact with the people closest to you and smile. If they don't smile back, shift your gaze so it looks like you were smiling at someone behind them.

Step three Now—and only now—walk inside, a slight smile still playing on your lips, and head straight through the center of the room. Even if you do end up standing in a corner, people's first impression will be one of confidence because you initially headed for the center. Got that mastered? Now, let's make sure you stay the center of attention by understanding the basics behind how to…

BE THE PERSON EVERYONE MOST WANTS TO MEET

Call it charisma, charm, or (more accurately) the ability to work the room, but people who've got "it," share more than a few common characteristics. The most popular person is more than likely to…

- **Look intelligent** You can usually tell if someone's bright or not, simply by looking directly into their eyes. People who aren't as bright, tend to have flat, lifeless eyes. Our eyes reflect the

> # Average, ordinary, nonthreatening people are approached **much more often** than extraordinary people because they aren't **seen as threatening.**

  activity behind them—when the brain is firing on all cylinders, there's more than a hint of things happening in our irises. Intelligent people are also focused—they're able to concentrate on a task and give it full attention. For this reason, their eye contact tends to be direct, unwavering, often intense. When intelligent people talk to you, they talk just to you—they're not the look-over-the-shoulder-for-someone-better types (unless you're boring them to death—the cardinal sin for bright sparks). Another sign someone's clued up: they walk and move quickly. Ambition often walks hand in hand with intelligence, which means setting high goals and wanting to accomplish a lot in life. They're rarely stop-and-smell-the-roses types.

- **Look friendly and approachable** We tend to feel more comfortable approaching people who aren't "too" anything: too good-looking, too ugly, too weird, too fat, too thin, too old, too loud. Average, ordinary, nonthreatening people are approached much more often than extraordinary people because they aren't seen as threatening and are less likely to reject our advances. This means being blessed with something fab—like enormous breasts or a stunning face and body—can backfire big time. If you're "too" something, including a little too gorgeous, it's even more important for you to…

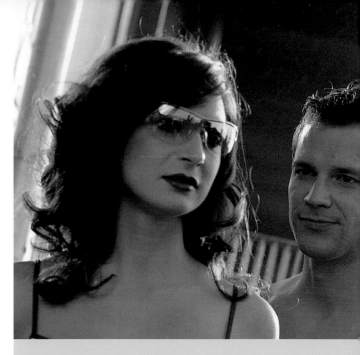

- **Give the green light to come over** If we want someone to approach us, we do several things: look directly at the person, smile, and turn our body toward them. If someone is doing all three to you—looking at you, facing you, and smiling—they're officially open to being approached.

- **Have relaxed and open body language** The person standing with folded arms or holding their bag or drink as a shield in front of them, doesn't exactly look welcoming. The person most likely to get chatted to (and hit on) has their arms uncrossed (hanging loosely by their side or in another relaxed position), stands with legs apart rather than clamped primly together, and their body turned toward the crowd.

- **Have their thumbs on display** Dominant, assertive (usually interesting) people invariably have their thumbs sticking up/out/on show. In palmistry, the thumbs denote strength of character and in body language, they're also a sign of superiority. Confident women will often leave their thumbs out when they put their hands in their pockets. Guys will often fold their arms across their chest, fingers under their armpits (often handily propped under a bicep, making it look bigger than it actually is), both thumbs left out on their chest and pointing upward. It's a conflicting signal— the folded arms are protective, the thumbs-up gesture shows confidence—but overall, it's interpreted positively. While we're on the topic of hands, it's not a bad idea to keep an eye on which way yours are turned if you're trying to impress someone. If you can avoid it, try not to turn your hands so that the back of your hand faces them. Our open palms and wrists are not only more aesthetically attractive, they're a sign of honesty and openness.

Instant sex appeal

There's another way to get yourself looked at—oooooooze sex appeal! Need a few tips on adding some oomph? Try any (or all) of the following:

- **Instead of dressing to cover up body parts you don't like, dress to show off the ones you do** You'll approach clothes shopping differently and end up with much sexier outfits.

- **Act the part** Relax your dress sense and body language and give yourself permission to be sexy.

- **Bypass your brain** Think about the person you most lust after. Imagine them sprawled, waiting for you on the bed. Naked. Begging for it. You've got one hour with them and no one's ever, ever going to find out what you did. DON'T let your brain think about practicalities, just give in to the fantasy. We're talking lust here, not long-term. Think fling. Better still, think flingette. The next time you're out and on the prowl, say to yourself "sexy thought" and connect with that feeling. If you feel like sex, your facial expression alters, you hold your body differently, naturally rearranging it to look its most attractive, and start emitting pheromones. Instant sex appeal, on tap!

Countdown to confident

Here's the really good news: you can transform yourself from shy to looking confident in about 60 seconds. There are five body language fix-its that will instantly make you appear more assertive—and the more confident you look, the better the response you'll get from people, and the more confident you'll feel. It's a win-win situation.

Before we get into specifics though, I want to say something. Being shy isn't something to be embarrassed about. We're all shy in certain situations, some of us just cover it up better, that's all. I walked into a meeting recently with my tummy doing more backflips than an Olympic gymnast. I felt incredibly nervous and shy—but I didn't look it. And that's what this is all about: teaching you how to cover up shyness and get you through the bit when the butterflies feel more like a colony of bats doing the can-can. It's the initial part that's the hardest—just about all of us eventually calm down and feel OK given a little time—so that's what we'll concentrate on here.

Why are some people shy and others not? It usually has a lot to do with our upbringing. Confident parents breed confident kids simply because they expose their children to more people. If your home is overflowing with neighbors, friends, and family, you quickly learn the basic social skills of how to interact with strangers, and make and keep friends without even trying. If you haven't had practice in the skills needed to turn an acquaintance into a friend, it's no wonder that meeting strangers is daunting. The solution to beating shyness is to mount a two-fold campaign: work on raising low self-esteem (which tends to go hand in hand with shyness), and interact as much as possible with as many different people as possible. If you don't feel capable of doing this yourself, get help. There are lots of books, workshops, and counseling opportunities to help nudge you along a little. While you're working on the inside, let me help by working on the outside and also give some practical advice on how to talk to strangers. Right! Now, let's go back to the five instant fix-its.

The first fix-it is to breathe I know, you're heard this one before "Take a deep breath, blah blah blah." Well, how about doing it? Because the first thing anyone does when they're feeling nervous or shy is to hold their breath. (The giveaway: taking very deep breaths occasionally, in an attempt to inject oxygen fast!) If you take a deep breath before speaking, it not only relaxes you, but it also gives you time to think. Another plus: it lowers the tone of your voice, making you sound more authoritative.

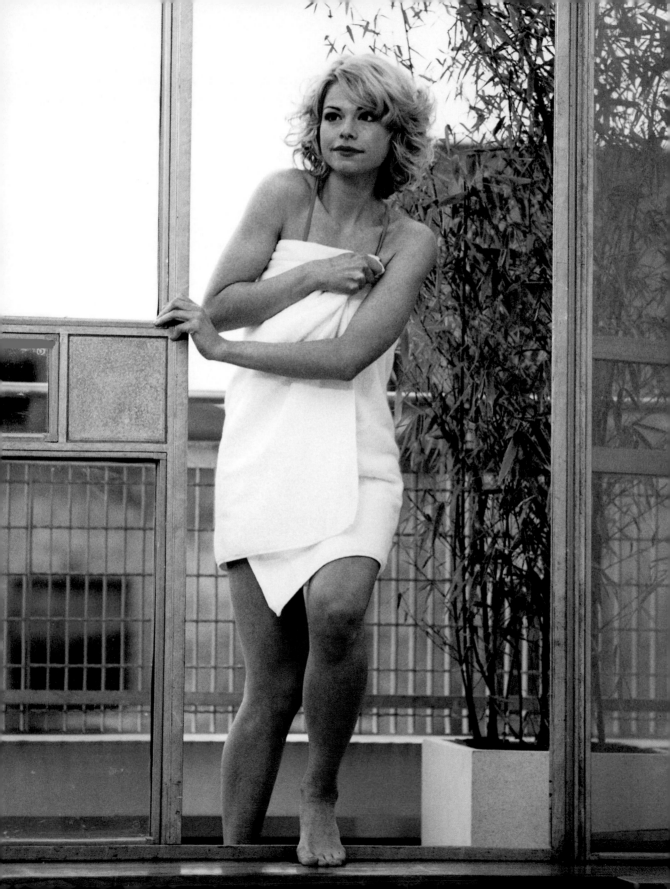

How to **take** a compliment

The first rule for taking a compliment: don't fish for one or you'll end up floundering. "So what's the best sex you've ever had," I once asked an old boyfriend, settling back comfortably and waiting for the praise. He beamed. "Oh, without a doubt it was this Danish girl. She was fan-tastic." Get the point? (I certainly did). Besides, a compliment delivered after a prompt is a bit like someone saying "I love you" when you've just asked, "Do you love me?" It doesn't exactly make your heart or head swell does it? Never mind other parts.

Compliments aren't **ping-pong balls**, you don't have to **keep serving** them back and forth

Now we've gotten that out of the way, the rest is easy. Because there's only one thing you really need to do if someone gives you a compliment: smile and say thank you. Then simply continue with what you were doing or saying. People (women) find it difficult to do this for fear of looking vain. If we simply say "thank you," isn't that like agreeing with them? Won't they think we're—deep breath now— a little too, well, happy with ourselves? This is why many women launch into that ridiculous "Oh, this old thing…" routine which does nothing except a) turn us into a cliché b) insinuate they've got bad taste. If you want to say something more, try "Thank you. That means a lot to me that you think that." Or "Thank you. It's really nice of you to notice." Another common trap: feeling you have to immediately compliment them back. "You think I've got great hair, well, hello! Yours is far nicer than mine." Resist the urge. Compliments aren't ping-pong balls, you don't have to keep serving them back and forth.

Fix-it number two Stand like a confident person: pull your tummy in, lift your chest to the ceiling, and square your shoulders by pulling them up to your ears, then back and down. Now, put your hands casually on your hips and make sure your body is directly facing the person you're talking to. This says "I'm giving you the best possible direct view of me because I'm happy with who I am and what I look like". (I know, inside you're cringing, but this is all about externals, remember?) One final adjustment to the way you're standing: shift your weight so it's on one leg. A study of business executives showed 75 percent of high achievers will assume this pose— hands on hips, weight on one leg—within half an hour of you meeting them. Practice the pose in front of a mirror until it starts to look natural, then pay attention because fix-it number three is the most important of all.

Fix-it number three The single, most effective way to change people's perception of you as shy, is to meet their eye. Easier said than done? Try this exercise: instead of looking at the sidewalk or downward, look straight ahead instead. That's a step in the right direction. From there, work up to glancing over to people's faces for a split second. Then, for a count of three, look at the tops of people's heads—you're not meeting their eyes, but looking vaguely at a point just above their forehead. Next step: imagine their face is a circle and travel around it with your eyes. Then concentrate on the features—mouth first, nose next, then (finally) focus on their eyes. Depending on how shy you are, it might take anywhere from two days to a month of taking baby steps to work through this exercise. There's another great trick for the really, really shy which means you don't ever have to make eye contact. Yes, really. Instead, make nose contact. Concentrate your gaze on the bridge of someone's nose instead of their eyes: very few people are able to spot the difference.

Once you're able to meet people's eyes, practice making eye contact with as many people as possible—three strangers a day, minimum. That's your target. When you're up to three people a day and you've done that for three days running, it's time to focus deliberately on people you find attractive. Now aim to make eye contact with three people you find attractive three times a week, then three times a day. Remember, you don't have to talk to them just yet, so it's not too stressful. Just make eye contact and, if you can possibly manage it, accompany that with a smile. That's more than enough to get you started and well on your way to the next part of our program: talking to strangers.

Fix-it number four Make yourself look safe to talk to. I don't mean put down the machete and remove the hangman's mask, just look friendly, approachable, and happy in your skin. Make sure your body language is open. Uncross everything. Don't hunch your shoulders. Don't frown. Lift your head up. That's better. Now, get yourself into position…

Fix-it number five If you don't naturally look confident, mimic those who do. By imitating their speech, style, and posture, you literally feel what it's like to walk through the world in their shoes. This is a great way to unlock their body language secrets, helping you adopt new confidence and learn new ways of communicating with people. When you find a gesture you like, adopt it as your own. About the only things you shouldn't mirror are negative body language gestures or particularly odd ones. If someone sticks a finger in their nose, ear (or elsewhere), they're on their own.

How to **give** a compliment

If the no-no for taking a compliment is don't ask for one, the don't-even-dream-of-going-there equivalent for giving a compliment is don't say it if you don't mean it. The second piece of advice: if you are going to give a compliment, make it as personal as possible. Ditch the "nice outfit" for "Your eyes look amazing against that gray top." Think of what you'd like to say, then substitute another word for the obvious. What's a better, more specific adjective than pretty/nice/smart/great? Also steer clear of the obvious body parts ("Gosh, you're tall!") and hone in on detail ("Haven't you got beautiful hands/lips/an infectious smile). But most of all ask yourself: what is that person most proud of?

A compliment, said **behind our back** often means more than **one said to our face.**

Another great technique is "accidental adulation": slipping praise into an otherwise bland sentence. Almost like the compliment slipped out. "This probably won't interest you but my sister's on this great diet…" (implication being you don't need to go on one). Passing on a compliment that someone else has made also works well for everyone involved. They're pleased, they instantly think more of the person who originally said it (a compliment said behind our back often means more than one said to our face), and you seem nice for passing it on. If you're far too shy to compliment directly, this is one way of doing it: tell a mutual friend instead and let them repeat it. It makes you seem less sycophantic and is a surprisingly effective way of letting someone know they're admired and appreciated.

MAKE CONTACT

Stand close enough to the other person to strike up a conversation, but not so close that they've got no choice. Then catch their eye, smile briefly but brightly, wait a second or two for a response, then look away. If they smile and make direct eye contact, they're open to talking. If they avoid your eyes and give a tight, closed-mouth smile, they're going to be hard work (shy or not interested).

SAY SOMETHING

I positively refuse to write list after list of suitable opening lines for every given situation. I'm not being a cantankerous old bag, you really don't need them. If there's one thing I want you to absorb from this

How to talk to strangers

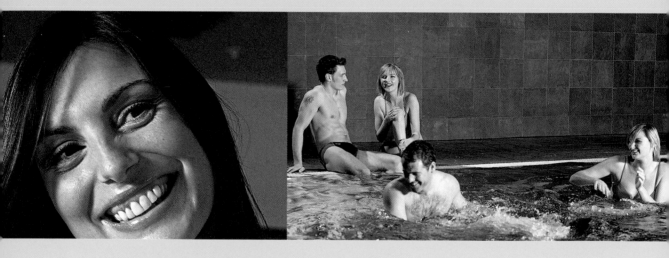

chapter it's this: pickup lines don't work. Visions of sleazy men in suits with greasy hair and gold chains pop instantly into our heads. The best pickup line is simply one that's appropriate to the situation you're in, and that's not too challenging. If you're in a deli and standing in line next to the best thing since sliced bread (sorry, couldn't resist), you're going to sound like a complete twit if you come out with, "You look like an angel who's dropped from heaven." Better to say, "Have you eaten here before? I can't decide between the chicken and the tuna." The more ordinary the topic, the better.

WHAT IF MY HEAD'S EMPTY?

Can't think of anything to talk about? The first lesson in journalism school is to answer five obvious questions in the first paragraphs of any story—who, what, when, where, and why. It's even more effective as a model for an opening line. Run through the five words and one's bound to inspire you. You're at the opening of an photography exhibition? *Who are you there with/to see?*—"Hi I'm Tracey. Do you know Wendy or are you a fan?" *What are you doing?*—"We've got the same cocktail. I've no idea what's in it but it tastes lethal." *When did you get there?*—"Did you get caught in traffic? I am always late." *Where are you?*—"These paintings are fantastic, aren't they?" *Why are you there?*—"Are you a fan of Wendy's work? I'm a friend, but it's OK to be honest. She likes constructive criticism."

WATCH THEIR REACTION

If they're happy to continue chatting, their smile will get bigger, they'll move closer and lean toward you. Don't give up if they don't instantly drip with enthusiasm: if you worry, you're far more likely to interpret shyness as arrogance, rather than anxiety. Other people get nervous too, you know!

KEEP IT GOING

Once you're happily chatting, move it forward from polite chit-chat to a real conversation by adding "feel" and "tell" questions. "Tell me why…" "How did you feel when…" If this doesn't get things

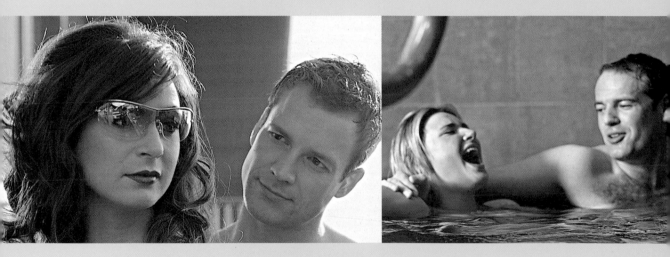

flowing (in all senses), the other person's either not interested and refusing to be drawn out, or you're asking too many "closed" questions. Open-ended questions need explanation ("What do you think of this place?"), closed questions can be answered with "yes" or "no" ("Do you come here often?"). Above all, keep smiling. Everyone likes people who appear to like them. Look like you're enjoying chatting with them and they'll be much more likely to enjoy chatting with you.

ARE THEY WELL-MANNERED OR GENUINELY INTERESTED?

If someone's chatting out of politeness, they'll take the first chance they can to end the conversation. Test them on this. Come up with a plausible excuse to leave their side for a few minutes and see if they're eager for you to come back. "I'm going to get a drink. Would you like one too?" If they're interested, they'll say yes even if they don't want one. Assuming you're not trying this pickup at an AA meeting, they'll say no if they aren't interested. '"That's OK, I'm going that way myself" or (the dreaded words), "I think I'll wait until my partner arrives." Damn. All that effort for nothing.

Exploring outer space
When and how to approach someone

Can you tell, just by looking at someone from a distance, who wants to meet you and who doesn't? You betcha! Whether they're splashing in the pool or waiting for the bus, everyone sends secret signals, giving all kinds of clues for the canny.

Proxemics is the study of how people use the space around them to send nonverbal messages. Most of us are more familiar with the term "personal space"—coined by a US psychologist in 1969 to describe the "comfortable separation zone" people like to keep around them. We carry personal space with us wherever we go, jealously guarding its boundaries and discouraging others from entering except by invitation or under unavoidable circumstances, like in a crowd. How much personal space we need depends on our country of birth, upbringing (touchy-feely families vs. prim and proper), personality, and experience. Introverts hold others at arm's length, preferring, literally, to keep an eye on them. Extroverts, usually the products of touchy-feely families, love the company of others, so like to keep them close. Which is why watching the two meet and relate is highly amusing: the extrovert steps forward, the introvert steps back, the extrovert steps forward, and so on. Each is trying to maintain the personal space that feels most comfortable to them. Culture also makes a difference. If you're from Italy, a country where people touch a lot, you'll stand a lot closer than the average Brit. The same applies if you were brought up in the city rather than the country. The closer you stand to someone, the more populated your home town tends to be. The more space you're used to, the larger the zone you'll keep around you as "yours."

As a rule of thumb, most people have more personal space in front of them than to their side. The least personal space is behind our backs. Like most things in life, personal space is…well, personal. In general, this is how it usually works: our social zone is around 4 to 12 feet. This is the distance observed by the relative strangers we interact with—the mail carrier, store clerks, the person working out beside you us the gym. Our personal zone is between 18 in and 4 feet, the distance we'll stand from others at parties and social events. We might not know these people, but they've been given some sort of approval so we trust them a little more. Our intimate zone (6 to 18 in) is the zone guarded most ferociously. Only those who are emotionally close and intimate—or those we'd like to be intimate with—are allowed here. As a rough guideline, these distances work a treat. But even without knowing the specifics, most of us figure it out, since we tell people how much space we need. Watch people at work—the person who spreads their belongings across the conference table wants lots of room to work. If we need to share a table in a coffee shop (and God, don't you

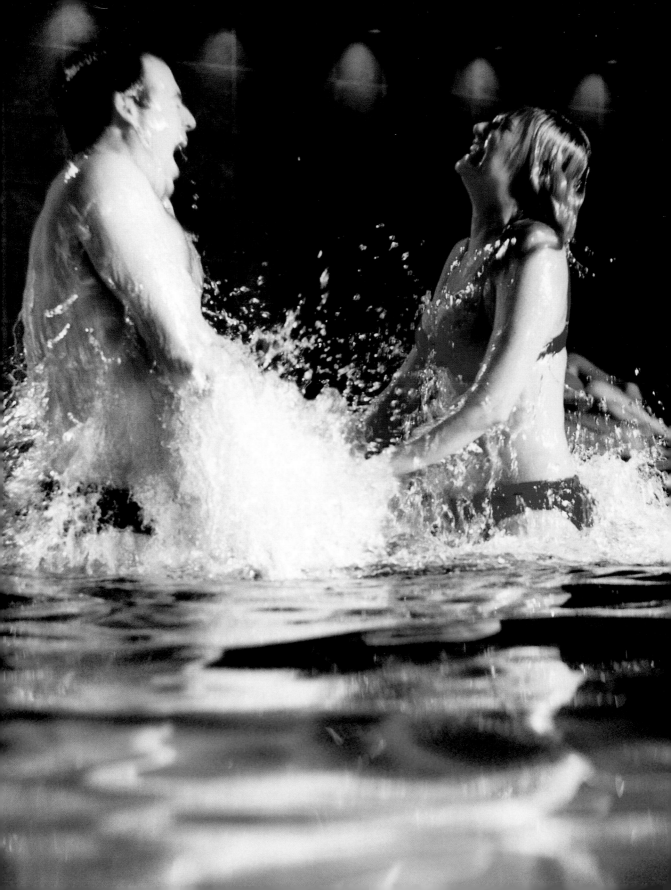

hate it?), we'll choose someone who's kept all their belongings neatly in front of them and left the other half of the table free. Space also indicates status. The more space someone needs, the more powerful they appear. Who gets the biggest trailer on a movie set? The star, of course!

So how do you know who's open to having their space invaded—and what's the best way to do it? A lot of it's logical: if we like someone or are attracted to them, we're much happier to let them stand closer to us than people we don't like or aren't attracted to. Different approaches also work better for different sexes. Women are more likely to be receptive if a guy approaches from the front. It stems from our primitive instincts: someone who approaches from behind or from the side could be about to hurt us. The prime flirting position for a man is to sit diagonally opposite a woman—one reason why dinner is a popular date choice. Historically, men attack men—and it's usually full-frontal. This is perhaps why a man perceives a woman who approaches him from the front as potentially threatening and challenging. She's better off approaching from the side and then moving around to face him.

If you want to invade someone's space, it's also a good idea to ensure that your eyes are on the same level. The person standing has the power, so if you want to be invited to sit down, lower your eyes to meet theirs. Test that someone is comfortable with the moves you've made to enter their personal space by stepping backward and seeing if they close the gap created. It's pretty obvious if you've invaded someone's space and they really don't like it. They'll step back or immediately place a barrier between you—a newspaper, bag, or glass of wine, and failing that, their arm. They'll also stand very still, their muscles will tense, and if they're forced to touch you, they'll do it on the least sexual part of your body (shoulder, elbow, clothed arm, or back). Get out of there!

COMMON QUESTIONS, PRACTICAL SOLUTIONS:
Q: The person I'm thinking of approaching just straightened up. Is this good or bad?
A: They've just squared When we see someone we like, we naturally "square" our bodies: in go our tummys, out goes the chest, we try to look taller and generally spruce ourselves up a bit. If someone squares when you look in their direction, there's a good chance they want to meet you.

Q: What are the signs a person isn't interested in meeting new people?
A: They're blocking We block to keep people in—and to keep them out—by using our body (or other objects) to establish a boundary around ourselves. Those we want with us are kept within the inner circle, others are warned off by barriers erected to mark our territory. We block using arms, legs, shoulders, and body positions, with chairs and bags, by the placement of beach towels or deckchairs, and by "bagging" seats at a function by putting our coats and/or possessions on them. We also block to stop others from claiming what we believe to be ours. A favorite pose of a sexually aggressive man is to put one arm up on the wall behind his target, effectively trapping her against the wall and under his arm. He's attempting to create privacy and gain her full attention so he can slip into superseduction without interference from others. The end result, unfortunately, has her fainting more from claustrophobia and underarm fumes than from passion.

Q: The person talking keeps closing their eyes and keeping them shut. What's going on?
A: They're doing what's called an eye cutoff or shutout This usually means they're stressed or nervous. Some people close their eyes when it's too painful to see what's going on; others do it during discussions or arguments in an attempt to shut out all stimuli and concentrate on what they're saying. Unfortunately, it also effectively cuts off any chance of their message being absorbed or sympathetically accepted by the listener because there's no eye contact backing it up. Bar interrupting—which is incredibly difficult to do politely when the person can't see you make "I'm about to interrupt" warning movements with your body—if you're on the receiving end of the shutout you're effectively cut off from communicating any response because you're not being seen. Not surprisingly, most people interpret the cutoff as insulting and unattractive.

> # **Women** are more likely **to respond** if **a guy approaches** them from the front…She's better off **approaching him from the side.**

Q: I've noticed a man across the room looking. How can I tell if it's curiosity or attraction?
A: It all depends on distance So says US body language expert Jan Hargrave. The screening line is the point where someone first notices you—around 20 feet away. If he's checking you out from this distance, it's nothing to get excited about. It'll take him 30 seconds to process whether you're his type or not (It takes women three seconds!!). If he's attracted, he'll probably keep staring until he gets closer. In the time it takes him to get to the attraction line—about 5 feet away—he's deciding whether he wants to meet you and how to orchestrate things. To buy time and think about what to say or do, he'll often slow down, maybe even veer away from you slightly to increase the time before the moment you meet. If he doesn't like you, he'll walk fast and walk past without looking at you again. The finish line is crunch time: he's beside you and unless he does something, all is lost. Even if he's too scared to make a move, if he's interested he won't be able to stop himself from stealing a look at your face close-up and will probably attempt to make eye contact.

Q: If you're attracted to someone, is it better to make eye contact from afar or up close?
A: For both sexes, it's a good idea to look from a distance Simply because it's less humiliating to be rejected from afar than up close. If they don't meet your eyes from across the bar, your chances of them looking thrilled to see you beside them are pretty slim. If you're a girl trying to pick up a guy, it could actually work in your favor to keep your distance initially. If he spots you at the screening line, it gives him time to process decide if he's attracted and what to do about it. If he sees you first at the attraction line, all is not lost, says Hargrave—but he will probably follow a set format. First, he'll give you a "stranger look"—a 1–2 second onceover, simply

acknowledging another human has entered his visual zone. He'll usually look back a second time, simply because he's clocked you're female. Now—and this is crucial—if he's interested, he'll look back a third time. It's the third look that's crucial: if he's given you three looks and is standing within 5 feet, you're in. Either that, or the sales assistant who convinced you that bright green kaftans are in was wrong. If you're not in a confined space—like a club or a bar—and he doesn't notice you until you're virtually side by side (at the finish line) you've got almost zero chance of meeting him, even if he is attracted. Why? Ego. He'd have to act extremely fast to register attraction and act on it in a split second, and few men have the courage to do an about-face and run after you. It's too humiliating. (One way to save this if you're interested: hold his gaze for as long as possible, with a definite smile. That way, at least he's been given the green light to come back). The short answer to the initial question: it's better to position yourself so he notices you from a distance. He needs time to process information and gather courage.

Q: I'm about to meet my new partner's friends. How should I approach them to make sure they like me?

A: First up, recognize they're as scared of you as you are of them As the new love interest, you're pretty powerful, too—you might monopolize his/her time so they never see them or decide his/her friends aren't good enough. Worse, they might prefer to hang around yours instead. If they're true friends, they'll have just one agenda: if you make your partner happy, they'll like you. If they're suspicious for some reason, you'll get clear signals. Protective friends will hug your new partner hello like they've been apart for years, not days—this means "We love him/her dearly. Don't hurt them." Telling lots of "in" jokes and constantly referring to the great times they've had, often means they're nervous you're going to monopolize his/her time. They want you to know a strong friendship exists and you're threatening it. The best way to combat that one is to laugh at all their stories, ask lots of questions, and act just as thrilled at their closeness as they are. The absolute no-no when meeting your partner's friends is to hang on too tight. It's a natural reaction: you're feeling threatened and the temptation is to seek reassurance by whispering "Do they like me?" into their ear. Don't. Having private little chats and separating them from the group is exactly what their friends fear. The only thing that would annoy them more is getting sulky if they're not hanging all over you. Yes, it's nice if they show affection so the group gets the message you're a couple, but pouting and flouncing around if they don't won't earn you brownie points with anyone. Instead of clinging, aim to be seen as your own person. Make an effort. No matter how unwelcome the reception, speak to each and every one of the group, if possible, starting off with a compliment ("Jane/John said you had the most amazing eyes and they were right" or "Jane/John absolutely adores you. I've been dying to meet you".) The best way to disarm outright hostility is to continue being nice, no matter how many darts are thrown your way. If, for some reason, the entire group seems against you, look for the person who seems the most sympathetic, take them aside, and say "I realize you're all very good friends with X and I just want you to know, I think the world of them. I'm looking forward to getting to know all of you and hope we'll have lots of good times together". If that doesn't work, wait until you get your new partner alone and ask some questions. They've

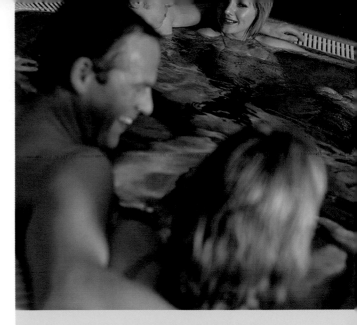

either a) got a habit of picking partners who put their hearts through a blender (leaving friends to pick up the pieces) b) have recently split with someone the group adored and want back again or c) have chosen friends who are utter bastards/bitches. If the last applies, get outta there fast. We can be judged by the company we keep.

Q: I always feel awkward joining a group of people if I'm on my own. Any tips?
A: Knock with your body language first

One of my favorite UK relationship experts, Susan Quilliam, has lots of tips for this one, all based on this idea that you knock with your body language before barging in. Start by standing just outside the group but reasonably close, smiling in their general direction. If they're open to newcomers, someone will eventually smile and move over to let you in. Once you're in the circle, make yourself part of the group by doing whatever they do. They laugh, you laugh. They look serious as they discuss politics, you assume the same expression. In other words, don't aim to make an impression initially, just be there and let people get used to you. When you feel comfortable enough to speak, look at the person who seems to be in charge. (If in doubt, simply choose the person doing most of the talking.) Make eye contact, tilt your head slightly to show you're listening, then raise your eyebrows. This hints you've got something to add to the conversation. When you do get the chance to talk, let your eyes travel around the group to include everyone and don't overdo it—this isn't the time to launch into a 10-minute diatribe about your mother's hip operation. Actually, it's never a good time, but especially not now. As the newcomer, you're expected to take a submissive role for a little while. If all seems to be going swimmingly well after 15 minutes, you can relax a little—looks like you've been accepted!

Once **you're in the circle**, make yourself part of the group by doing **whatever they do.** They laugh, you laugh. They **look serious** as they discuss politics, you assume the **same expression**.

Eyeing up the talent

From lowered lashes to wicked winks we communicate more with our eyes than any other part of our bodies. Not surprising then, that eye contact is the ultimate flirting tool. Get this part right and the rest is easy.

A wink saved my life once. Well, my self-esteem anyway. It was the first time I'd returned to London after my parents emigrated to Australia and a friend of mine had put me in touch with a friend of his, who'd generously offered to let me stay. Christopher lived in Wimbledon and turned out to be incredibly "posh." He was also funny, sexy, generous, and all-around gorgeous. Which somehow made it even worse when he insisted that I join him at a never-ending whirl of society functions. A 21-year-old student, my suitcase wasn't exactly bursting with Versace originals, so I was forced to show up dressed in bizarrely inappropriate things. I remember standing awkwardly in a group at the Ascot races, convinced I was committing all manner of social sins (and was, apparently), feeling gauche, unsophisticated, shy, and painfully out of place. (You try wearing Doc Martens and a miniskirt surrounded by a sea of designer dresses). The only time I looked up was to steal a quick glance at Christopher, to see if he felt as embarrassed at me being there as I did. But instead of looking humiliated, he gave a sexy little smile and a big reassuring wink. In the blink of an eye, he'd said "I know how you feel, but you're doing fine. I'm here with you, relax." That wink was devastating. It made me feel accepted, sexy, admired, reassured, and downright fantastic. It made me lift my head up, square my shoulders, meet the eyes of the person standing next to me and strike up a conversation. I went from having the worst time of my life to the best time.

In a tense situation that one small movement of the eye had a dramatic effect, and when you consider that 80 percent of our information about the outside world comes through our eyes, it's hardly surprising that almost all dating experts rate eye contact as the ultimate flirting tool. Eighteen times more sensitive than our ears, our eyes are capable of responding to one and a half million simultaneous messages. So finely tuned, they'll subconsciously spot when someone starts looking at us and start taking mental notes. If that person is checking everyone out, they'll stop registering the information; if it's just us they're interested in, they'll signal the brain to give us a nudge that someone's watching. (Forget the earth mother image, Mother Nature is a complete and utter sexpot!) Vital for communicating all emotions and particularly handy for interpreting sexual signals, it's hardly surprising this entire book is littered with references to eye contact techniques.
Turn the page and find a few to get you started…

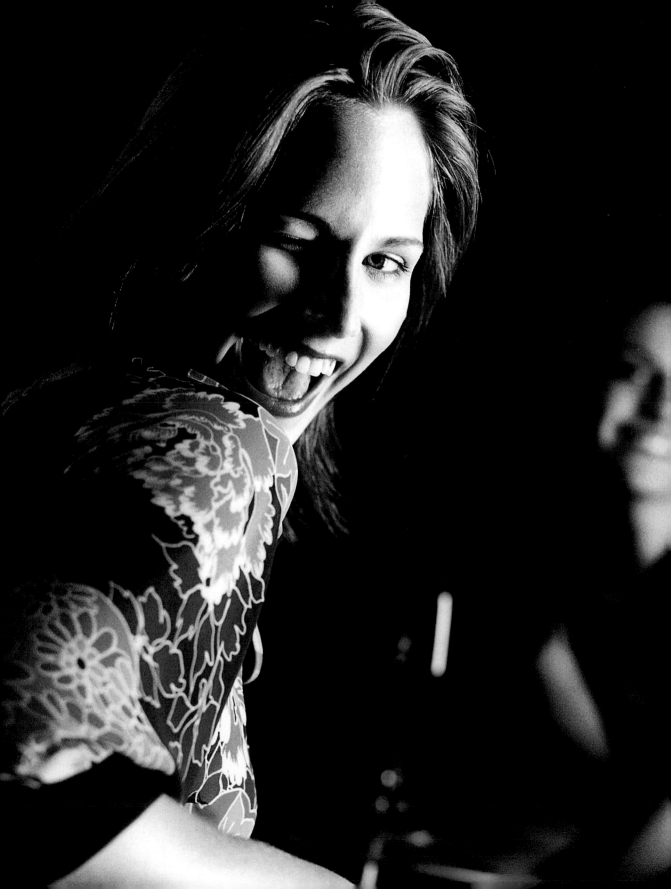

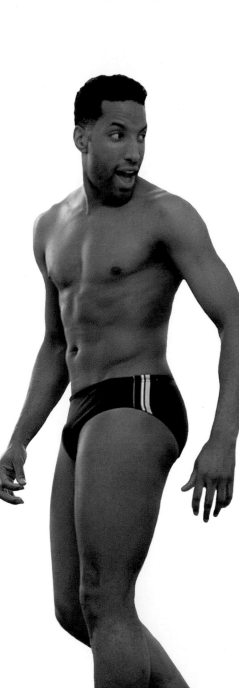

- **Focus attention** Draw attention to your eyes by using something to point to them. Our eyes automatically follow movement, so by pushing your hair away from your eyes or by tapping near them with a pen, you'll force anyone talking to you to look up and into your face. Another quick trick: put your thumb underneath the side of your chin and rest your first and index fingers on the side of your face pointing toward your eyes. (An added bonus: not only will it draw attention to your eyes, it subliminally makes people think you're intelligent because you're pointing to your brain as well.)

- **The four-and-a-half second scan** A normal face scan lasts three seconds; scan for four and a half and it's clear they've "caught your eye." Eye contact of more than 10 seconds between two people means one of two things: you're about to fight or have sex (well, you want to anyway). Prolonged eye contact produces intense emotional reactions regardless of whether it's a fist or a pair of lips heading your way. It activates the nervous system, raises the heart rate and blood flow, and stimulates the production of certain hormones. Just about everyone knows being watched is a sign someone's interested, so if you want to subtly make your intentions known, this is the way to do it.

- **The slide and settle** Let your eyes settle on someone so they're aware you've noticed them, then as they're still watching you, slide your eyes around the room before settling back on them again. This effectively says, "You instantly attracted me and you're still the pick of the room, even after I've checked out the competition." One other point while we're on the topic of eye slides—if you're interested, it's best to break the very first eye contact made by dropping your eyes straight down, then directly up again to lock eyes after a few seconds. If someone's eyes instead slide away from yours to the side or upward and don't return after a minute or two, they're almost definitely not interested. The slide and settle is a quick movement—the whole thing's over in 10–15 seconds—but it's impressively accurate.

- **The flirting triangle** Eye movement studies show we look at different parts of other people's faces depending on the situation and level of attractiveness. When looking at strangers or in business situations, we make a small triangle by moving our eyes from eye to eye, dipping them as we move across the bridge of the nose. With friends or in more friendly social situations, the triangle widens as our eyes drop below eye level to include the nose and the mouth. With lovers and people we're attracted to, the triangle broadens even further, dropping below the mouth to include the breasts and other good parts, like the genitals. The more intense the flirting, the more concentrated the eye contact becomes at certain parts of the triangle. Eye to eye contact becomes fast, furious, and constant, seconded by long periods spent staring at the mouth. Our eyes spend the rest of the time making little side journeys to the parts at the bottom of the triangle.

- **Blink if you're interested** It's easy to see where the term "batting your eyelashes" originated from: if someone looks at us and likes what they see, they tend to blink more. Because the brain associates rapid blinking with finding someone sexually attractive, the more you blink at someone, the more attracted you feel to them. This, of course, can be manipulated to your benefit! You can increase the blink rate of the person you're talking to, by blinking more yourself. If the person likes you, they'll unconsciously try to match their blink rate to keep in sync with you, which in turn, makes you both feel more attracted to each other! Don't automatically assume slow blinking means disinterest, however. If we're completely absorbed in a task, concentrating or addictively entertained, we blink very little, not wanting to miss a second of what's before us. Confused? Don't be. Common sense and other body language signals will tell you which interpretation applies to your situation.

- **…and wink if you want more** As evidenced by my little story, a quiet wink matched with a sexy smile can be incredibly bonding simply because it's secret and implies the two of you are closer than others present.

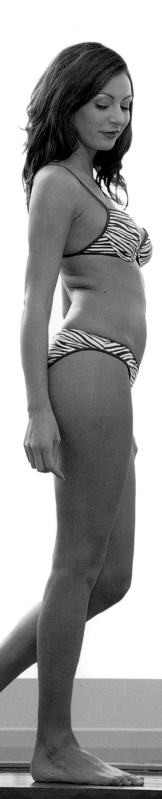

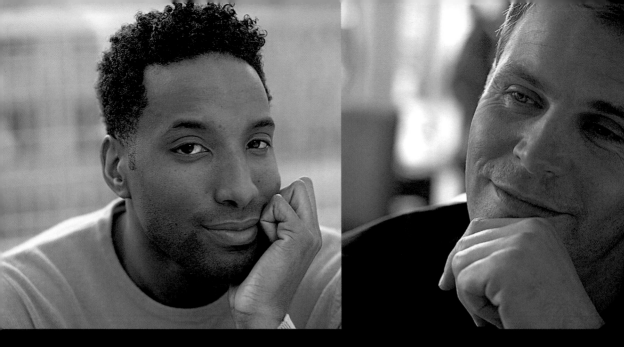

Hand signals

Our hands are one of the most expressive parts of our bodies, offering endless clues on how we're really feeling. Here we see examples of boredom (a typical pose is the hand on chin, top left), interest (an evaluation gesture, top right), self-confidence (church steeple, opposite), sexual interest (hand pointing to genitals, bottom left). Clasped hands (bottom right) can be a neutral gesture (loosely knitted fingers) or indicate frustration (fingers gripping tightly).

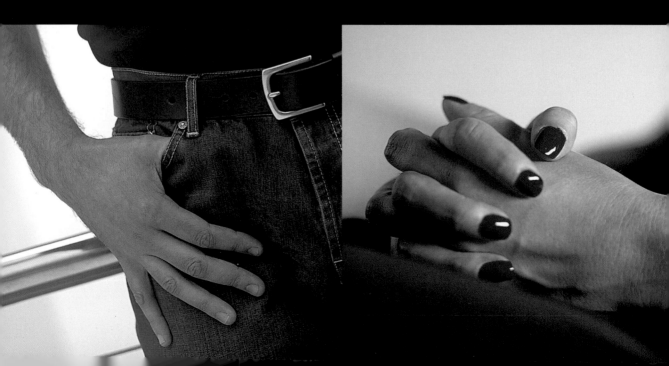

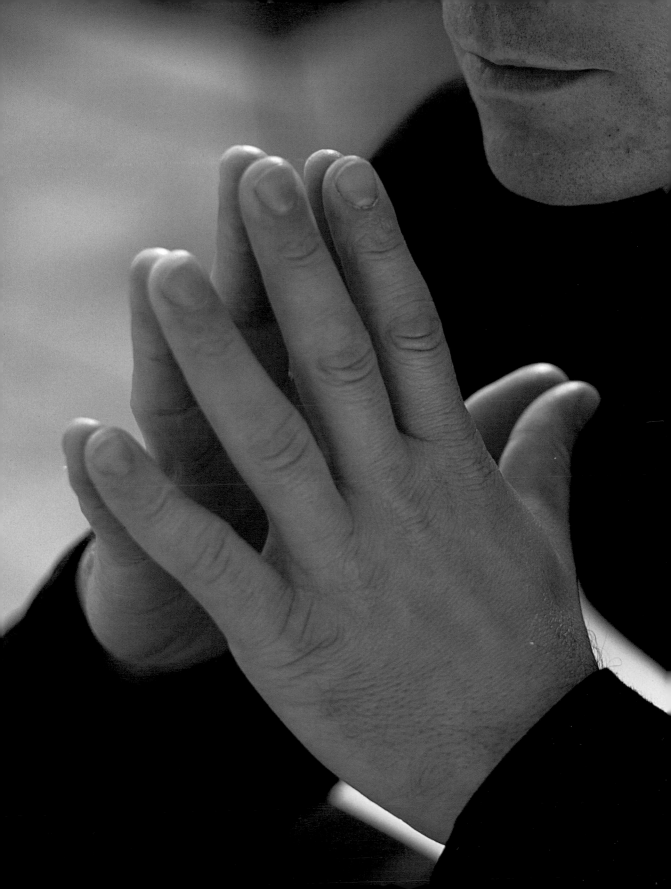

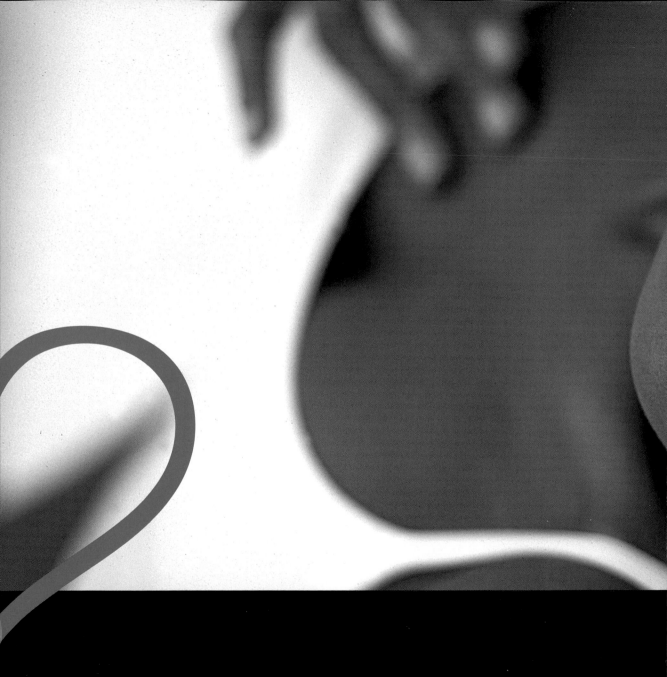

SEX IT UP

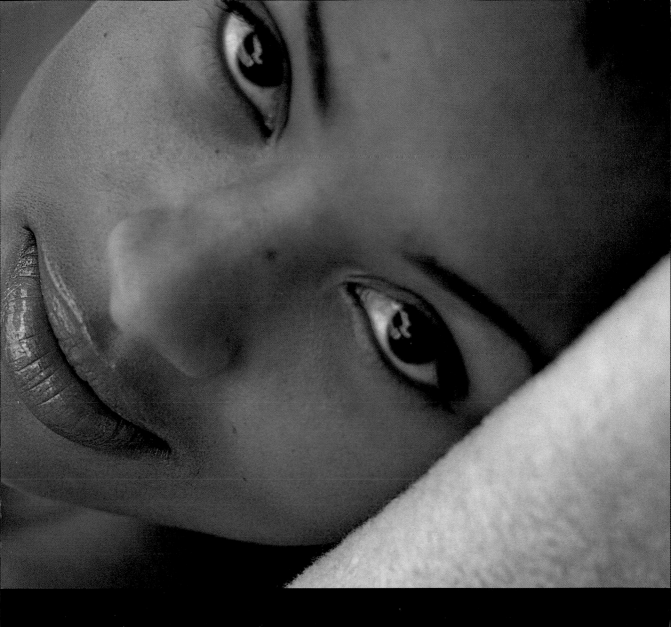

Turn up the vamp volume with a do-it-yourself sex makeover; spot the three different flirting styles; and **transform from so-so to supersexy** in the blink of an eye!

How to make yourself sexy...

The 13 secrets of sex appeal

What makes someone sexy? Good question! After all, what's sexy to one person is "Are you kidding?" to another. I'm not entirely sure whether it makes me sad, hopeful, or a resourceful workaholic (it's my job, after all, to work with potential), but I can usually find something sexy about practically every person I meet.

As evidenced by one (admittedly, rather bleary) morning standing outside a hotel in Bordeaux while waiting for the rest of the crew to get their act together—and trying hard not to be seduced by the upmarket shop windows—I got seduced by the sight of a man sauntering up the street toward me. The French really have got that sexy look mastered, I thought to myself. I mean, look at this guy! The slightly disheveled hair, the shirt buttons undone, the deliberately unshaven look. It's all so well done, it's a little contrived really, I sniffed…Except…what was he doing rummaging around in that garbage can? I know there's probably a law against being attracted to tramps, but it is a compliment, and it does illustrate my point. Sex appeal is all about attitude and aura and making the best of what you've got. This guy wasn't waiting for money or status or society's approval before he'd let himself feel sexy. He just was—and being seen rummaging aroung in a garbage can didn't stop him from throwing me a killer smile and saying something which sounded deliciously naughty. (Who knows what he said, quite frankly, but it sounded guttural and gorgeous.)

Of course, what people really mean when they ask "What makes someone sexy?" is "Am I sexy?" and "How can I be sexier?" So let's just get right down to it, shall we? Here are the real secrets of sex appeal, along with how you can use the evidence in a practical way to boost your sex appeal.

1. Both sides of you match The more symmetrical your face and body, the more sexually attractive you are, and the more attention you get. It's not the result of nasty brainwashing by society either—even babies go ga-ga for symmetry. Far more manipulative than the media is Mother Nature. She consistently protects the health of the species by making sure that those from the strongest gene pool (in this case, the symmetrical) are seen as the most attractive. While no body is ever truly symmetrical (so stop stressing about your left boob/testicle being smaller/lower than the other), appearing "matched" helps immeasurably. Female bodies are actually programmed to appear 30 percent more symmetrical on the magical high-conception day after ovulation. People with symmetrical bodies usually lose their virginity much younger and have more sexual partners than their lopsided friends.
Lesson: Wear matching socks. (Not much else you can do to influence this one.)

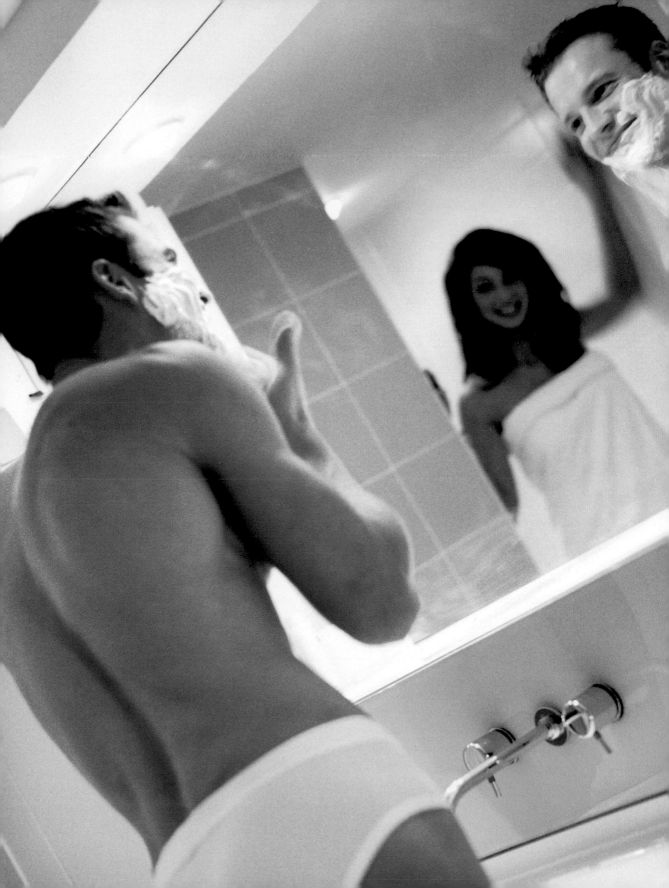

2. You look like your genitals Err, perhaps I'd better explain this one. Sex-obsessed creatures that we are, anything that reminds us of sex usually gets us going. A female with full, glossy, red lips is a turn-on because her lips mimic what (he fantasises) is happening elsewhere: the vagina also "plumps," moistens, and darkens in color when aroused. Phallic-shaped foods like zucchini and bananas also subconsciously influence desire. Which goes a long way towards explaining why a) hotdogs are so popular (let's not even go there about the sauce), b) people cling to the myth about oysters being an aphrodisiac, and c) the "just got out of bed" look never goes out of fashion (we like to imagine anyone attractive in one—with us of course). In the same vein, a "fertile" face is seen as a beautiful one. Clear, fresh skin, shiny eyes, youthful, plump lips, a cold nose—a healthy-looking face like that tends to come attached to a body which is bursting to conceive. That's right, good old Mother Nature again, guiding us to the people most likely to keep the planet populated!
Lesson: Feel zero guilt when spending big on lip gloss, and load it on.

3. You've got a big mouth Researchers created computerized versions of the average female face before getting test groups to rate their attractiveness. The first set were awarded an average attractiveness rating. In the next set, researchers increased the eyes and lips by 10 percent. The result? The faces were seen as younger and more beautiful. Once these features were exaggerated further, the faces were universally judged as sexier. Look at the makeup on a typical model: lots of heavy eyeliner to enlarge the eyes, full lip gloss to accentuate the lips. Exactly the look you should aim for if you want to inspire lust…and if all you're searching for is a short-term fling. If you're after a long-term love affair, then a totally new set of rules apply! Bury the "all men are bastards" theory forever (it's ridiculous anyway!): it's personality, not looks, that men go for in a long-term partner. A sexy face might inspire lust, but it's the girl with the average face and nice personality who hooks up long-term. Why? It's her again! Men choose women whose idea of heaven is staying at home to raise their babies rather than dancing half-naked on a podium.
Lesson: Looks count, but it's your personality that makes people stick around.

4. You walk young Along with swinging hips and general "attitude," there's another crucial element to harness if you want to be seen as sex-on-legs: flexibility. Flexibility is what makes people appear to "walk young"—an instant winner in the sexy stakes.
Lesson: Loosen those limbs.

5. You make pots of money Countless studies show women continually go for good looks and money and if forced to choose between the two, money wins every time. I strongly objected to this research, convinced it was inaccurate. I'm not money-obsessed and neither are my girlfriends, so I asked a broad selection of men (between the ages of 15 and 80) what the real story was. I'm embarrassed to report they all said this is true of 80 percent of the women they meet. I'd rather believe it's the old baby theory again (he earns enough to support you) rather than greed.
Lesson: Money is the root of all evil…blah, blah, blah

6. You look like a girl, even though you're a bloke Just like a man, the type a woman goes for depends on what she wants from the relationship. This was nicely illustrated by an experiment which allowed women to control the features on a computer-generated face. By moving a bar, they could make the man's face more masculine or feminine looking. Most of the time, the feminine face won their hearts because they trusted and felt safer with this look. During ovulation, when women are at their most fertile, the sweet guys didn't get a second look. To hell with nice, they all said, this is about sex, and they pushed the bar in the other direction to choose the most masculine face possible. Post ovulation, when lust takes a backseat and logic settles in, the women again rejected the masculine men. Then they were voted too aggressive and womanizing: "a man like that would want lots of sex and seek it elsewhere if he didn't get it at home."

Lesson: The message for both sexes is clear: we're attracted to one type of look/person for sex, another type/look to marry. Customize yours to suit.

7. You score on their sexual lovemap We're attracted to people who look or act like other people we love or have loved. From the moment we're born, our brain continuously feeds us physical data about people close to us. It divides these characteristics into "people I like and were nice to me" and "people I don't like who hurt me", then it tries to generalize. If two-thirds of the people you've disliked had bushy eyebrows, you'll be suspicious of everyone who has a hair or two extra. If it was the opposite, your tongue will be on the floor at the sight of them. When we meet a potential partner, our subconscious checks against the "liked people" list in our heads and tries to find the closest match. The more

A female with **full, glossy, red lips** is a turn-on because her moist lips mimic **what (he fantasizes)** is happening elsewhere.

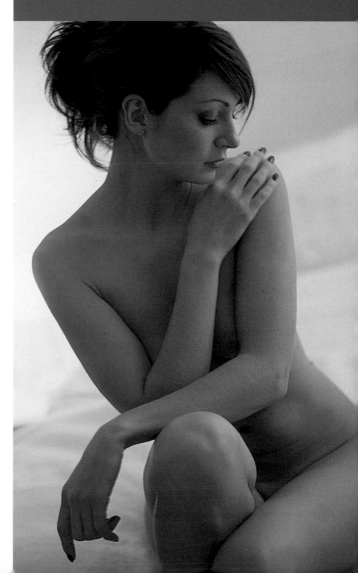

"chemistry" we feel, the more matches we've found. We do the same with gestures. The way she brushes the hair from her neck, the dimple he gets when he smiles, all affect our opinion of who's sexy, who's not.

Lesson: Don't take rejection personally. It's not just about you, it's about their past. (All the more reason to take risks and go for what you want!)

8. You stick your butt out Women spend their lives worrying about the size of their buttocks—yet the more pert and rounded they are, the stronger the sexual signal. Females of all the other primates send sexual signals via the color and smell of their buttocks, which, since they walk on all fours, are in full view of potential mates. To show your butt off to its best advantage, turn your back to someone you're attracted to, put your hand on one hip, shift your body weight so the hip with your hand on it juts out farthest, then turn your upper torso around and make eye contact. Just as good: put your hand in the back pocket of a tight-fitting pair of jeans or (absently) slide both hands over your hips. The overall show-off-your-bottom award though goes to…high heels. Heels lengthen legs and shorten butts. The average increase in the protrusion of a woman's buttocks wearing heels is 25 percent. (This, remember, is a good thing.) They might not have their own ass-index, but a tight, toned male bottom also rates extremely high on the "whoa!" sex scale.

Lesson: Stop asking "Does my butt look big in this?" and start asking, "Does my butt look big enough?"

9. You've perfected one supersexy look The best look I've ever received was from a guy sitting opposite me in a restaurant. His eyes slid up, caught mine and then, maintaining eye contact, he sat back, put down his knife and fork, and simply stared at me. His lips curled in a half-smile that made me drop my eyes to look at his mouth and that's when he caught his bottom lip with his teeth, released it slowly and then, when my eyes went back up to his, smiled. It wasn't a would-like-to-get-to-know-you smile. It wasn't even an I've-watched-you-watching-me" smile. This was predatory: a we-both-know-I-could-make-you-faint-with-pleasure smile. I suspect he was right because I damn near fainted on the spot, without him even touching me.

Lesson: Copy what he did or invent your own. Choose from the many eye contact techniques in the book, then add your own individual mouth, hand, or hair movements until you've come up with your own signature "sex look."

10. You've chosen your moment Certain events and situations make us more attractive to someone. If someone's just been dumped, lost their job, or been through a rough time, they're much more likely to find you sexy than when life's going well. When your self-esteem is low, you underestimate your own attractiveness and overestimate other people's. You're vulnerable, need a hug, and are less fussy about who gives it to you! Being scared also has the same effect—but for different reasons. Research shows that when our bodies are flooded with adrenaline, we're more likely to want whoever is with us at the time. Which makes mountain climbing or skydiving a damn good option for a date (though a roller coaster ride or seeing a good thriller will also do the trick).

Lesson: It pays to be around immediately before and after things like job interviews and dreaded public speaking events. If you're interested, volunteer to hold their hand.

11. You don't go overboard on the compliments Once, while making a TV show, I had to do multiple takes walking in and out of the front door of a busy bar. The first time I walked in, a guy sitting near the bar said to me, "I read somewhere that you're 35, but there's no way you are. You're having us all on." Given that I was 39 at the time, I was obviously flattered and the next walk was a hell of a lot jauntier. Problem was, he insisted on telling me the same thing

> The average increase in **the protrusion** of a **woman's buttocks** wearing heels is 25 percent. (This, remember, is **a good thing.**)

every time I came through the door. All 10 takes were ruined by his you-don't-look-your-age line. My suspicions were confirmed (and ego dashed) when another man came bursting through the doors to claim him. "He escaped," he said, "he's not meant to be unaccompanied". Excellent. You get my point though. When someone tells us we're sexy, young-looking, funny, bright—whatever— it has the optimum effect the first time it's said. Keep harping on it and you not only dilute the compliment, but you also get the opposite reaction to the one intended: instead of liking you, they find you annoying.

Lesson: Only compliment people once on each particular attribute.

12. They know you're attracted We like people who like us. If you know someone thinks you're fabulous, you instantly up their attractiveness to make it more of a compliment to you. It also forces you to consider them as a prospective partner and—perhaps most importantly— provides some (often much-needed) feedback. You've got to have hope or you give up. There's no point in being attracted to someone when you know without a doubt that there isn't a chance in hell of ever waking up to find their face beside yours on the pillow.

Lesson: Let people know if you think they're sexy.

13. You're happy to take your clothes off Few of us are completely happy with our bodies and proud to prance around naked. Yet nothing is sexier when it's let's-get-naked time than someone who shows off their wares and lets their lover admire them, rather than cowering under the covers.

Lesson: Relax about your body. Knowing you're sexy is a turn-on.

Tempting tresses

Hands up those of you who've never had a bad hair day? Sorry, but being bald doesn't count. The fact is, most of us are acutely aware of how much our hair affects our looks, but it also influences our personalities. And not just because a great hair day makes us feel instantly happier and sexier. People make all kinds of assumptions about us based on the style and color of our hair. There's little to support the stereotypes, but people continue to make them anyway. If you've got dark hair, you'll be seen as much more serious than someone who's blonde. Blondes score high on sex appeal, but not so great on intelligence or friendliness. If every redhead got a penny each time someone blamed an emotional outburst on their hair color, most could retire by 50. Short hair signals how strong, capable, and straightforward you are; grow it long and you're instantly sexier, flirtier, more vain and frivolous. There is some logic there: long hair does need more time spent on it, so a no-frills, no-nonsense person might just keep their hair short. Greasy, dirty, unkept hair sends a clear message of zero self-esteem (not to mention, makes us look slightly crazy!). We also tend to choose a hairstyle that reflects our personality. I once cut my hair off and hated it. Not only did I feel horribly exposed with nothing to hide behind, but I also felt a bit like Samson. He lost strength, I lost sex appeal. Don't get me wrong, I know lots of supersexy women with short hair, I'm just not one of them (don't even get me started about my profile). Most of all though, I missed having long hair to flirt with. It's a remarkably versatile flirting tool. You can toss it, flick it, peek through it, play with it, twist it, and run your fingers through it.

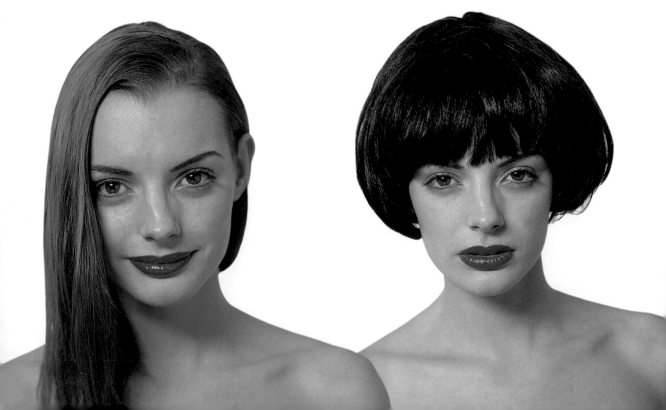

If you've ever doubted how much hairstyle influences personality and someone's perception of us, think about what happens to people when they put on a wig. Costume parties might be a pain in the butt initially (all that effort finding a costume), but you're almost guaranteed good gossip the next day because people behave out of character. Put on a wig and you pull on the personality stereotype that goes with it. You've got an excuse to be more outrageous, and to flirt with the person you wouldn't normally dare to. Grab a girlfriend, rent some wigs, and take yourself

> # Your lover's **taking you for granted?**
> # Put on a wig in a completely
> # **different style** or color and they'll **react afresh.**

out flirting for the night. If you're shy or lacking in confidence, your "disguise" could be just what you need to practice being a new, more adventurous you! Wigs are also fabulous for making people look at you afresh. Your lover's taking you for granted or you want to turn a friend into a lover? Put on a wig in a completely different style or color (flattering, of course!) and they'll react afresh, seeing you in a totally different light. Because you look like a stranger, all their natural attraction instincts revert to "first meeting" setting, which is when they're most likely to say whether they're attracted or not.

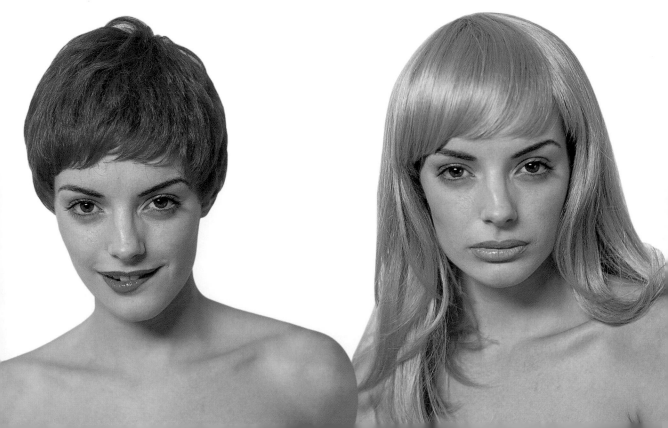

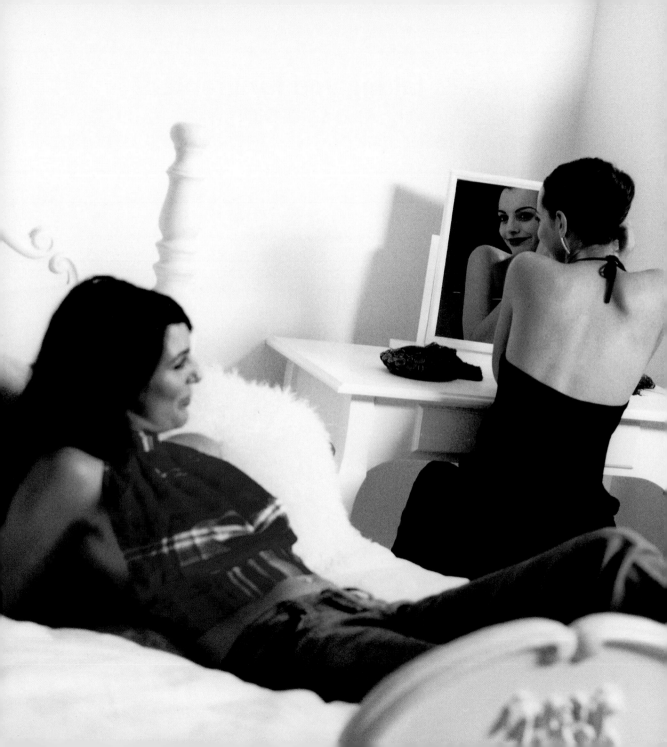

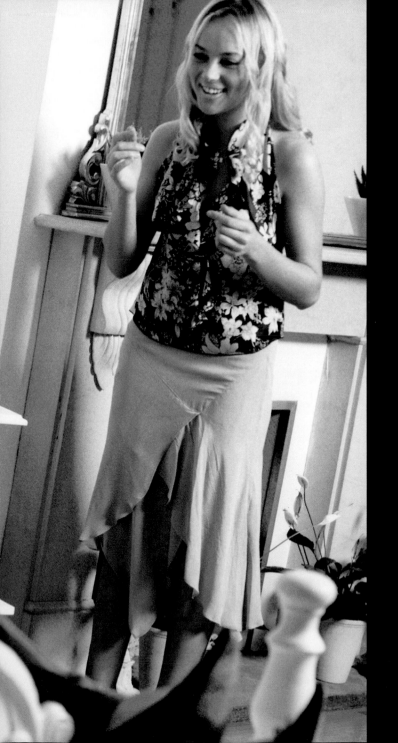

One glance at this picture tells you these girls have different personalities. What's also obvious—once you know what to look for—is their individual flirting style. The clues lie in their innate sensory preference: all three are represented here. Aural people prefer to communicate by what they hear; visual people by what they see; and kinesthetic people by what they touch and feel. We're all a mix, but one preference tends to dominate. That "I feel like I've known you forever" feeling we get when first meeting someone is because they hear, see, or "feel" the world the way we do. You both experience life the same way, so feel an instant connection. All isn't lost if the person you're attracted to isn't your "type," but you do need to tap into their world and speak their language to get them on board. (Say "See my point?" to an auditory person and you might as well be speaking in tongues. They don't "see" anything. "Hear what I'm saying?") How do you spot who's who? One of the most reliable indicators is the position of the eyes. Our eyes flick up, down, sideways, and left to right as the brain searches for information, each position activating a certain sense. Visual people tend to look up, to their imagination; auditories to the side, toward their ears; kinesthetics down, toward their heart. Pinpoint where someone looks and you're often set. To find out other surefire signals and why smiles are also a clue, turn the page…

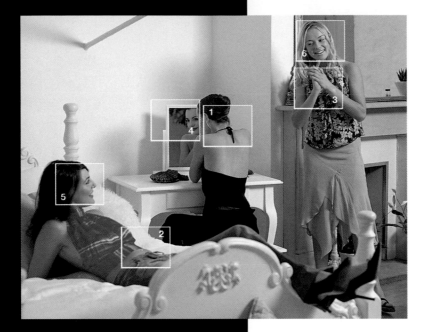

Can you spot the

Character clues

- **The best flirts take no chances and appeal to auditory, visual, and kinesthetic types. They'll cue words and actions to get people to listen, feel, and touch.**

- **Visuals tend to laugh the most and the longest. Which probably makes them the most chilled out, since one full minute of laughter relaxes us for up to 45 minutes afterward. It also makes them highly attractive: the ability to laugh out loud and make others laugh are key ingredients to sexual attraction.**

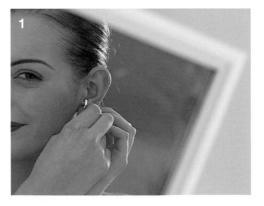

The auditory (1) Not only is she looking to the side as she listens, but she's also decorating her ears (naturally, she chooses earrings as her only piece of jewelry). What's not typical of her type, who make up just 15 percent of the population, are her clothes. Most As don't notice what they're wearing—the elegant style comes courtesy of Ms. V., who took her shopping.

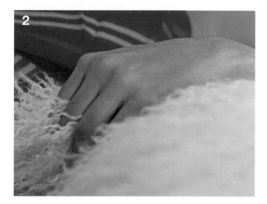

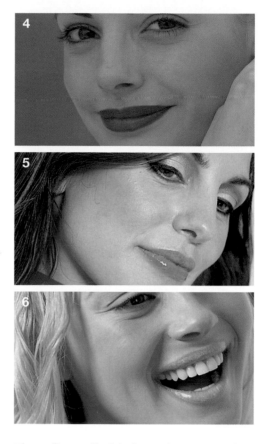

The kinesthetic (2) Kinos touch anything and everything, which is why she can't resist stroking the cushion. Her sexy outfit is true to type. Making up 30 percent of us, Ks are sexually experimental and hedonistic. What's not apparent is her sensitivity. Despite the vampy, "bad girl" image, she gets hurt easily.

flirting style?

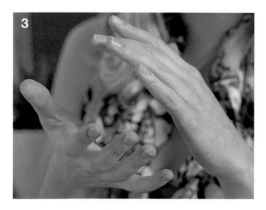

The visual (3) Visuals paint pictures with their words and, literally, by using their hands to "sketch." She's a fast talker and bubbles with enthusiasm, an earmark of her high-energy, visual personality (55 percent of us). The strongest clue however: her coordinated clothes. Vs like looking good, and it's obvious she's worked hard on her appearance.

The polite smile (4) The smile says Ms. V's story is wearing a little thin for Ms. Auditory. Her smile is tight and strained and it doesn't reach the eyes. Being analytical and logical, she can't see the pictures V's trying to paint.

The self-satisfied smile (5) While Ms. K is amused by V's story, you can tell by her smile she's distracted. The dreamy expression suggests she's thinking of something secret and special. Being a K, it's bound to be strongly connected to her feelings—a lover perhaps?

The genuine smile (6) Ms. V gives us a fine example of a "light up the room" smile. We can see lots of teeth, her head is thrown back to expose her neck, her lips stretch as broadly as possible, and the eyes twinkle and crinkle with happiness.

Like it or not, people will make assumptions about you simply by looking at the things you own and wear. The photos below show the possessions of the girls on the previous pages—Ms. Audtiory, Ms. Kinesthetic, and Ms. Visual. Can you tell which possessions belong to which girl? Here are some clues.

MUSIC

Most music collections reveal a theme (romantic, quirky, traditional, alternative). Sort yours into music styles and you'll instantly see the impression they're giving—most of us don't stray from three or four styles. Other collections are so eclectic in taste they completely confuse—the only conclusion you can safely reach in this case, is the owner has many sides to their personality.

What your **possessions** say about you

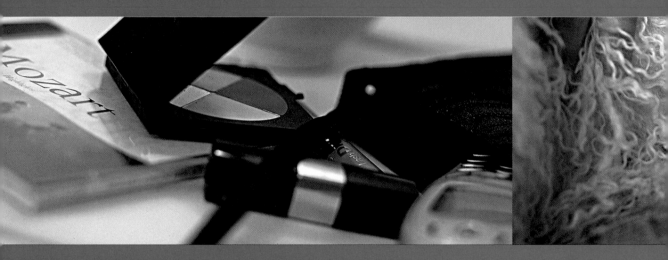

SLEEPWEAR

A cartoon-character nightie for her or striped PJ's bought by Mommy for him send a clear message: if you're invited to sleep over, snuggles and cuddles are all that's on offer. While few of us sleep in Victoria's Secret type underthings (even if we should), there is a middle ground between frothy wisps of nothing and flannel pajamas. Ironically, an old, seen-better-days (but oh-so-flattering, hence why it's worn to death) t-shirt often does the trick for both sexes.

TATTOOS AND PIERCINGS

Anything unusual but voluntarily afflicted on your body will stamp you with one of many labels. Choose from cute, rebellious, sexy, bad, urban, hip, attention-seeking, or vulgar, depending on who's doing the judging. Although piercings provoke a passionate response, they are removable and therefore not permanent. Tattoos are different. Almost everyone has a reaction to them, the majority voting no. I'm not saying they can't be sexy, but be aware the mark you make will be much more than skin deep.

JEWELRY

Highly individual jewelry also speaks volumes. Large, dramatic pieces go with big, dramatic personalities. Small, delicate, girly jewelry is chosen by traditional, feminine women. Those who wear heart-shaped pendants, earrings, or bracelets are nearly always romantics. Men wearing jewelry (other than the usual watch) make an even stronger statement. He's either cutting-edge trendy (bold silver pieces that are distinctly masculine), dreaming of a veggie burger eaten by the beach (beads hanging on a leather cord—the surfer/hippie type), or announcing his sexuality (he's gay).

SHOES

The shoes we choose reflect our personality and our intent as effectively as a mirror. Ever been picked up wearing a pair of sensible flats for a flirty night out with the girls? Didn't think so. High

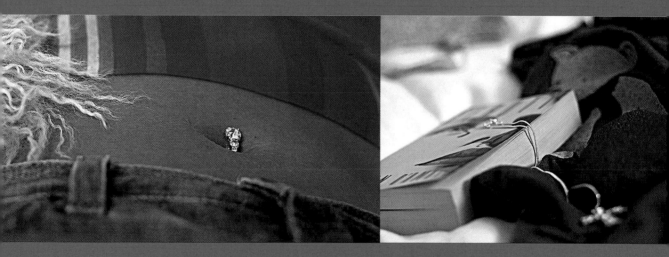

heels, particularly strappy ones, can be the epitomy of sophistication— or send out wickedly wanton signals. It all depends on the height. One-slip-and-you'd-break-your-neck shoes reek of sex because only a girl on the make would risk life and limb simply to look hot. Men have less choice in footwear but face the same type of dilemmas. Too shiny, overly conservative shoes make him look uptight and prissy, while scruffy old running shoes like he hasn't made an effort. Myth has it the more shoes you have, the more you long to travel and see the world. This is obviously why the average woman has 30 pairs stashed in the closet. Nothing to do with fashion at all. So there!

HOW DID YOU SCORE?

Did you guess who was who? Left to right they are: Ms. Auditory—note the classical CD and the chic mobile phone. The middle photo featuring the piercing and the hand running through the textured cushion focuses on Ms. Kinesthetic. Finally, the romantic novel, delicate pendant, and cartoon-character nightie in the photo on the right belong to Ms. Visual.

From frump to fabulous

Do you really believe you need to be beautiful to have them lined up and taking a number? Don't be silly! Research shows we're most comfortable with people who are similar in attractiveness to us. So you don't need to look like the latest heartthrob to be seen as sexy. In fact, it's the good looking who should be anxious.

People who are lots better looking than the norm make us feel uncomfortable. We're acutely aware of not measuring up and feel the scales are massively tipped in their favor— which makes us feel uncomfortable and paranoid and it's all too difficult, so why even bother going there?

Some of you will read this, breathe a sigh of relief, and (apart from a suspicious twinge of the too-good-to-be-true's) happily accept it. Others won't be able to. If your body image is particularly bad, you simply won't be able to make the connection between "good enough" and "my body." To say this is interfering with your sexual relationships—both getting one and enjoying it while you're in it—is the understatement of the millennium. Hating the way you look stops you from connecting to your sexual self, which stops you from feeling, and therefore appearing, sexy to others. How did you end up this way? Relax—it's sooooo not your fault! No one is born hating their body, we learn to dislike it in response to life experiences—and of all of these, our early experiences with touch are crucial.

It's virtually impossible to love someone and not touch them. You can't have sex without touch, and it's damn difficult to show affection and emotion without it either. Feeling comfortable touching others and being touched is vital: it's the foundation on which relationships are built. Whether you're a touchy-feely, can't-take-my-hands-off-you toucher or the don't-you-dare-come-near-me type, it pretty much all comes down to one thing: your childhood. More specifically, your family.

How our family uses touch is our testing ground for how we'll use it. If your Mom and Dad touched you frequently and lovingly, you've learned to link touch with love. Even better, if everyone in the family – Mom, Dad, siblings, grandparents, everyone—used touch to express other positive emotions as well (caring, support, and comfort, etc.). Assuming nothing traumatic has altered this, you'll have grown up to do the same. Sadly, not all of us are this lucky. Some parents' idea of a touch is a hit. Overanxious, clingy Moms leave us associating touch with being smothered. If you've grown up in a family whose touch is infrequent, when it does come it can feel more like an electric shock than a loving gesture.

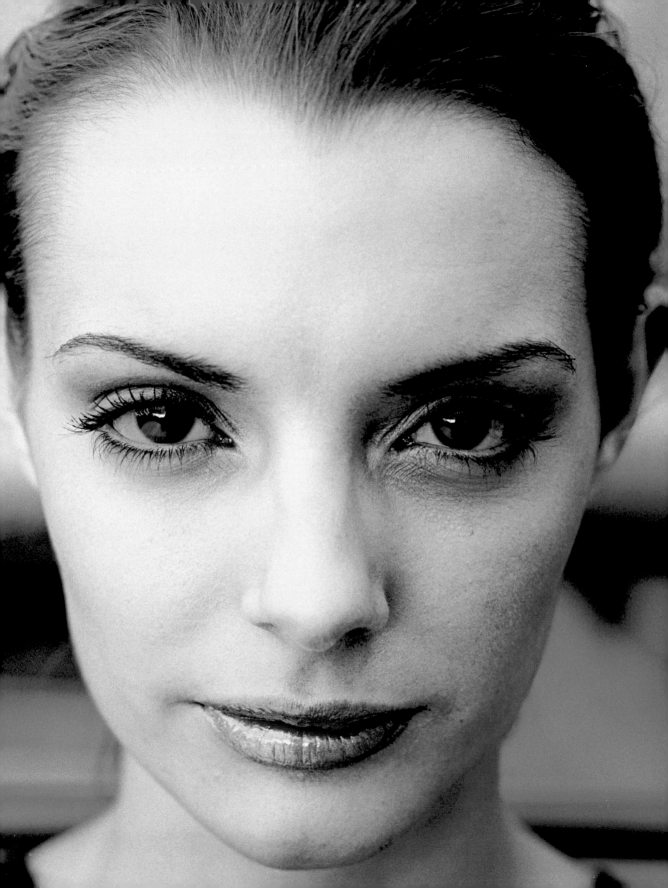

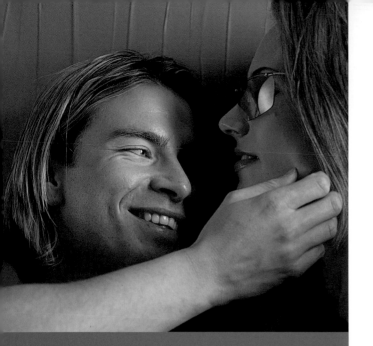

Touching in public

A word of warning for those who discover the joy of touching: keep an eye on the volume control. There's a tendency to be a bit too enthusiastic at the start. Most of us do a subconscious "appropriateness" check each time we touch our partner in public. An acceptable "public" touch would be putting an arm around your girlfriend's waist. An unacceptable touch, best reserved for in private, would be putting your hand under her clothes. Hundreds of other touches fall somewhere in between, with each couple and/or individual, rating the acceptability of each according to the stage of the relationship, their attitude to touching in general, and who "the public" is. The better the friends, the more "private" touches we'll make in front of them. Ironically, the less demonstrative you are in public, the more bonded you're likely to be. There's less need to prove your love to each other or to others and, usually, the longer you're together, the better you "read" them. Long-term bonding means you can communicate affection or adoration by myriad smaller, less obvious tie-signs (signals to show you're bonded). Sometimes, all it takes is a glance. So don't be too envious of that over-affectionate couple you know have been together forever!

If you experienced any of this as a child, you didn't learn to link touch with love. Which means as an adult, you've probably got no end of problems. Many studies have shown that when parents have failed to connect touch to pleasure and love, their children go on to have problems with romantic and sexual relationships later in life. Not being touched at all can actually be fatal. Studies of infants in orphanages show that unless they are touched lovingly by their caretakers, the babies become so depressed that they die. They literally give up on living and everything shuts down.

People who have touch problems are relatively easy to spot. Their personal space boundaries are bigger than football fields. Move forward to shake their hand and they'll move back so fast, they're practically sprinting. If you ever can get close enough for a hug, it feels like hugging an ironing board. Problems with touching often go hand in hand with body image issues as well.

We begin forming an opinion about our body— how we see it and how we think the rest of the world sees it—virtually from birth. This body image is sometimes nothing like how our body actually is in reality. (In a sense, how we feel about it is probably more important than what it looks like!) Our body image starts being shaped by how we're touched and held—lovingly or with zero affection—by our parents. The messages we get from siblings, friends, teachers, and peer groups shape it further. General attitudes via the media and society continue the job, and our lover's opinions about our bodies finish it off.

Loving, well-balanced parents manage to teach appropriate morals and modesty but also encourage a healthy curiosity of how each part works, simply by using the right amount of touch. The bottom line is this: if your parents weren't complimentary about your body or pretended you didn't have one, you're not going to be too pleased with it either. As psychologist Aline Zoldbrod says, in *Sex Smart—How your Childhood Shaped Your Sex Life and What To Do About It*: if no one in the child's world ever comments on how cute we are or makes any sort of comment about our physical appearance, we grow up feeling either invisible or unappealing.

The only thing that's worse? Insults. Even innocent teasing has a long-lasting impact. Never mind that you've grown up to resemble a stick insect, if your Dad nicknamed you "Tubby," tubby you may feel for the rest of your life. Throw a few playground taunts on top of that and you're an eating disorder waiting to happen. The criticism that we got as a kid tends to turn into the critical voices that whisper in our ears as adults. The ones that say "You're too fat for that" when we pick up a slinky dress and "They won't like you—you're too stupid" when we're struggling to flirt with someone. A bad body image wrecks our self-esteem and our relationships. For a start, it stops us from

> # If you don't like your body, you won't like people **touching you** and you'll feel uptight when it's on display. **Like in bed, for instance.** Being sexy isn't about bodies, **it's a state of mind.**

meeting people—you're not exactly going to dash across a crowded room to meet the person of your dreams if you think they'll take one look and say "Yuk!" Even if you get that far, it's difficult to believe someone else finds us sexy and attractive unless we believe it ourselves. Hurdle over that obstacle and you'll hit another: if you don't like your body, you won't like people touching you and you'll feel uptight when it's on display. Like in bed, for instance. The reality is that being sexy isn't about bodies, it's a state of mind. Regardless of body shape and size, if you dress, act, and think you're sexy, others will see you that way. If you've got serious body image or touching problems, I'd strongly recommend you take yourself off to a good counselor and work through them. If they're mild, try the following exercises. Some are adapted from Zoldbrod's book.

BEAT A BAD BODY IMAGE

- **Make a body map** to discover how you feel about touch. Draw two pictures of the outline of your body, one representing the front, the other the back. Imagine yourself in a pleasant and private situation with someone you love romantically. Then, using three crayons (red, blue, and green), color in the picture according to the following guidelines. Use red to color in places on your body you don't want to be touched under any circumstances. Blue means "It depends on

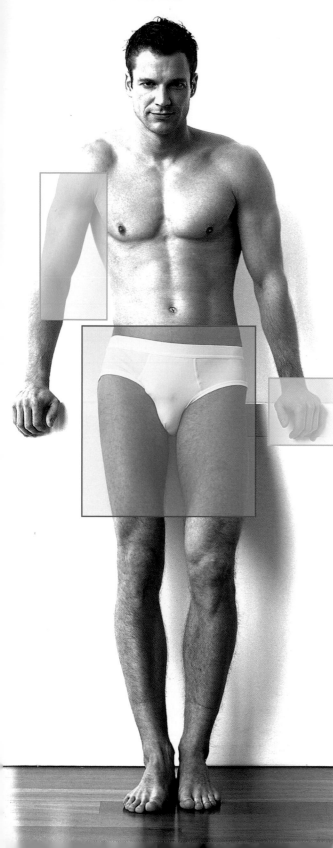

how I feel on the day whether you can touch me there." Areas you color green are places you don't mind being touched any time. Now sit back and take a look at the results. A healthy body image should produce a picture with mostly green, a small amount of blue, and virtually no patches of red. If there are "no-go zones" they're there for harmless reasons (your underarms because you're ticklish). If the opposite is true—there's very little green and lots of red, it's extremely likely your ability to enjoy sex is severely hampered. Try doing the rest of the exercises along with reading Zoldbrod's book (there are lots of other reading references listed at the back of her book), then repeat the exercise. If there's still no improvement, you might consider seeing a counselor or sex therapist.

- **Look at childhood photos of you and your family** They provide invaluable insights about the messages your parents gave you about touch by revealing who tended to touch who where, and in what way. Are your parents touching each other in most of the photos? Are they touching you? Do all the children get touched equally? Are you and your siblings touching? Ask a friend who you think is comfortable in their own skin and with their own sexuality to show you their family album. Compare the two sets of prints and I expect you'll start to see how you've each ended up the way you have. Understanding means you're on the way to solving the problem.

- **Join a dance class** Any will teach you to move your body in a sexier way, which boosts body confidence. Some—like bellydancing—openly encourage you to connect to your sexual self. Classes like ceroc and salsa involve lots of body contact, forcing you to get you used to touching other people. An added bonus: you never know who you might meet!

- **Get a pet** People with pets are happier, live longer, and have much lower stress levels than people without them. Stroking a cat or dog is one of the most therapeutic touching exercises you can do. Animals can teach us lots of lessons about touching. Watch a cat reward its owner for touching it: not only does it arch to meet the hand, but it also purrs approval and closes its eyes with bliss. No wonder you'll sit for hours, letting it lounge in your lap!

- **Ping a rubber band** This technique sounds overly simple (not to mention slightly whacky) but it's incredibly effective and adaptable. It involves wearing a rubber band around your wrist (tight enough for you to be conscious of it, but not so tight your arm falls off) and pinging it whenever you have a negative thought. Let's say you're a guy who got teased at school about being too puny and despite evidence to the contrary—muscles from weight-lifting and compliments from girlfriends—you still feel puny. Just wearing the rubber band helps because it shows you're attempting to rise above the paranoia (and by doing so, recognizing your problem might not actually be based in reality). Pinging the band—hard, so it hurts!—every time you hear a voice in your head say "puny" means your brain starts to associate pain with thoughts of being puny. Do it often enough and the brain eventually intervenes, taps you on the back, and says "Listen. Every time you think "puny," it causes me pain. So stop doing it OK?" And so you do.

- **Give yourself a hug** We often touch our own bodies to comfort ourselves. When we're little, our parents dispense hugs. Hugs aren't so easy to come by as an adult. The one person who is always with you wherever you go, however, is you. It might not feel quite as good as when a partner does it, but it's better than nothing.

Sexier in a second!

- **Act the part** My friend Emily is drop-dead gorgeous but hides inside severe business suits and tightly bound ponytails. We were at a bar recently when she sighed, "All the other girls get looked at. I never do". "That might have something to do with the fact that they wear tops the size of bras and skirts split to the waist Em. Your outfit's not exactly vampish, is it?" I said ruefully. "You want me to be more like they are?" she said, and started mimicking a girl who'd just sashayed past. Em's a great mimic—even with the suit on, she'd transformed herself into a sex kitten. "Umm, yes," I replied. "But I could never be like that. Not me." "What if you weren't you?," I suggested and dragged her off to the bathroom. Hair released from the ponytail, the first few buttons of her shirt undone, jacket removed, the only thing left to do was to yank up the skirt. She looked both horrified and mesmerized by the results. "We're doing an experiment. Get out there and pretend to be the girl you saw walking past." Up for a laugh, she did what I asked. Within 10 minutes, a guy came over to flirt with her. Lesson learned, Em's relaxed her dress sense and body language and given herself permission to be sexy.

- **Admit that change is good** Most people like routine and tend to fight any type of change. Our brains like our thoughts to be routine as well. When something happens to us, our mind compares new information with something similar from the past and looks for recurring patterns. It then predicts what is going to happen in the future. In other words, it tries to make similar life experiences end up the same way. This means if you always do what you have always done, you will always get what you have always gotten. Fine if you're happy with your life; not so good if you're not. Be actively aware of this, to stop the process from demolishing your chances of change.

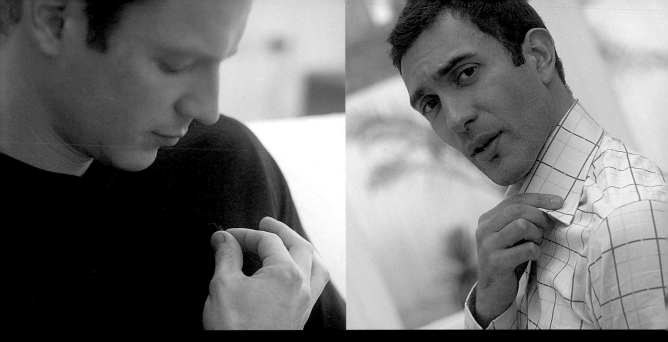

Preening gestures

We preen when we want to look our best and attract someone's attention. Men preen by straightening their collars (top right) and brushing or removing lint from their clothes (top left). They'll literally pull up their socks (bottom right) when they see someone they're attracted to. Women also adjust clothing, but more commonly play with and smooth their hair (main picture and bottom left).

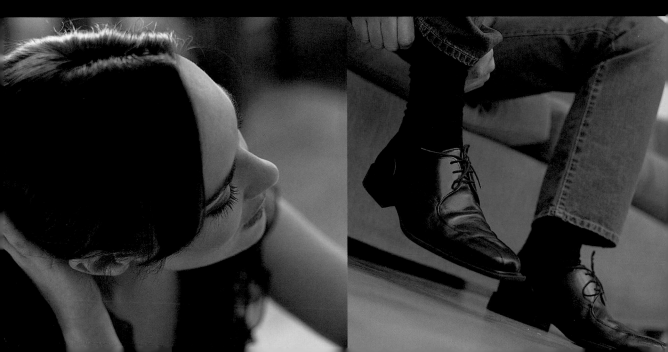

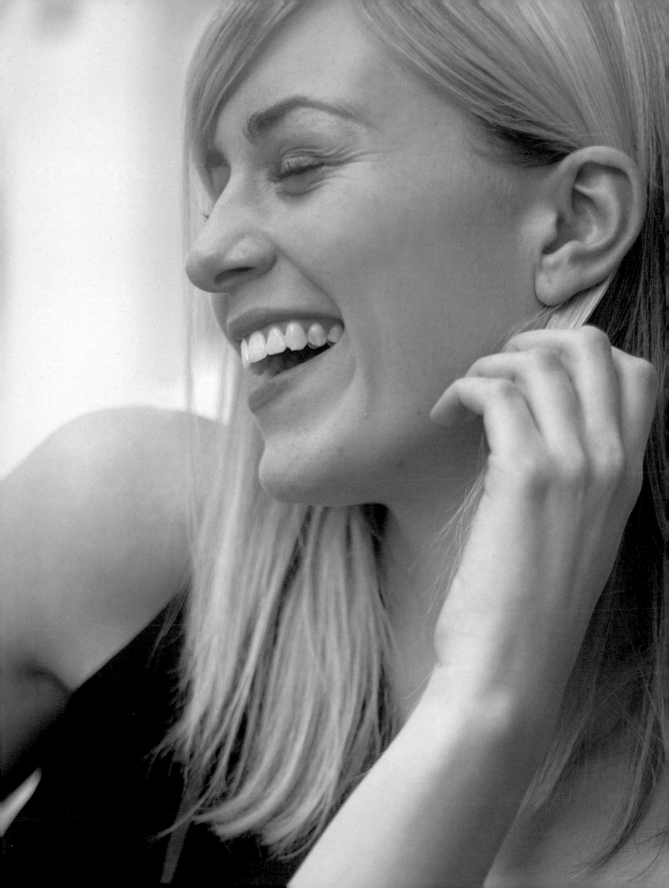

3

FLIRTING
FUNDAMENTALS

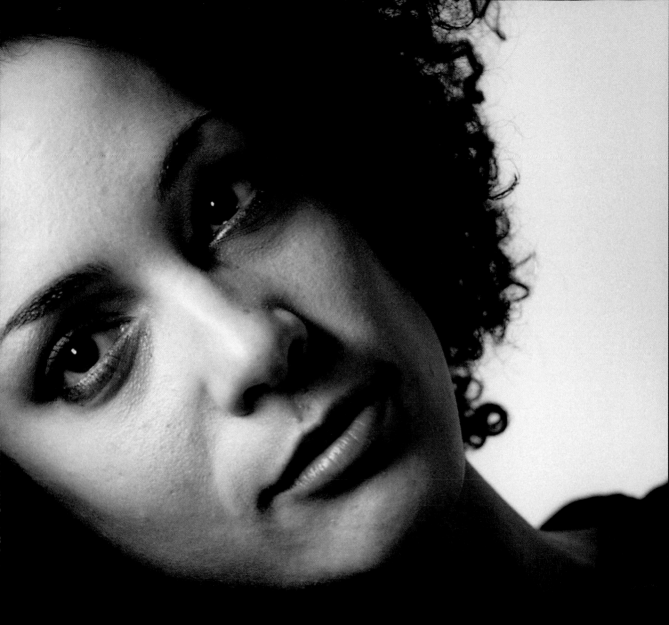

The foolproof signs they want to be (much) more than friends, fancy footwork, how to **figure out someone's personality** from the way they sit, and **why being a copycat** is a very good idea.

Be a babe magnet
Tricks to keep that little black book bursting

Batting eyelashes might beckon you over, but there's more to winning her over than simply crossing the floor. You need some sneaky, simple, and oh-so-effective ways to mesmerize from your very first meeting.

Superflirt is crammed with tips and hints on how to make yourself more attractive to women. Just in case you're not entirely satisfied, however, here are a few more.

THE PICKUP

- **Look for "shiny" eyes** If she's gazing up at you with twinkly eyes that seem to sparkle with excitement, she's probably interested. Chances are you've aroused her emotions— with a bit of luck, perhaps passion or adoration. Intense feelings cause the tear glands to secrete fluid, but if the emotions aren't intense enough to produce an overflow of tears, the liquid pools instead. Excess moisture causes light to bounce off the eyeball, making the eyes "dance" and look more attractive. It can't be faked either, so glistening eyes are a good indicator that you're having an effect on her. Be forewarned though: fear, stress, and discomfort manifest in exactly the same way.

- **Take a visual voyage** It doesn't matter who we are, if someone locks eyes with us for too long of a time, most of us feel like a butterfly with its wings pinned. Thing is, it's rather easy to become mesmerized when you're gazing at someone who's so damn sexy, you're practically drooling. Fix it by forcing yourself to feast on the entire spread laid in front of you— in other words, take a visual voyage. While you're chatting, take time to check out her cute nose, the curve of her cheek, neck, and shoulders. Hover around her hairline, look at her earlobes, caress her entire face with your eyes. The trick to making your target feel admired rather than minutely examined is to keep the visual voyages short—flick back to her eyes for long seconds in between. Later, when all systems are go and you're ready to move it forward into a kiss, it's OK—even desirable—to make it obvious that you're studying every part of her. On the topic of staring though…

- **Gaze, don't stare** Initially, a flirty "I think you're quite alright" look should only last the time it takes you to say the words out loud. In the beginning, you're playing a game of "I see you, do you see me too?," using your eyes to signal a quick expression of interest. (It's only later that longer periods of eye contact come into play.) Pay attention here guys, because this is when it can all go horribly wrong. Stares can easily be mistaken for glares, and there's a big difference between gazing and staring. When we gaze, our face is softer. Dreamy eyes, a half smile, slightly lowered eyelids all indicate that we're daydreaming about the person we're looking at. A stare is much harder: a set, stern mouth, lips pressed together, wide, unblinking eyes, and an unwavering expression all mean

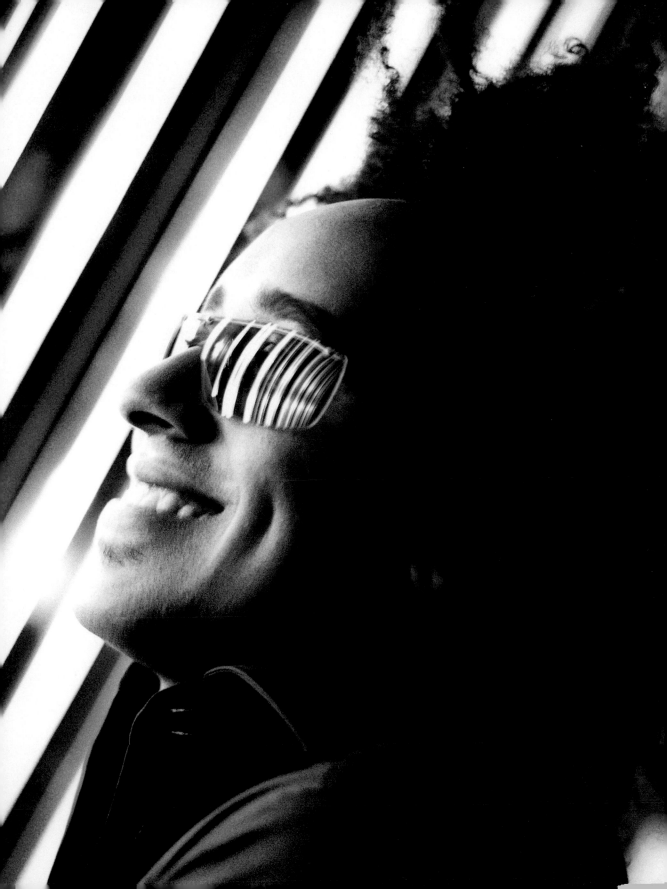

you're curious or fascinated by what you're looking at…but not necessarily in a good way. The thing is, what feels like a gaze from your end can look like a stare/glare from theirs because of our individual mannerisms and face shapes. If you're worried your come-on look is killing your chances, grab a mirror and see for yourself. If your gaze seems too hard, imagine you're looking at the person you adore most in the world and watch your eyes and face instantly soften, open, and relax. Restrict your gazes to no longer than five-second bursts until you're almost at kissing stage… then feel free to lock eyes (and limbs) for as long as you like.

ON A DATE

- **Value yourself** You know what it's like: you open a birthday present and instantly think "Yuk!". You'd asked for a new wallet and that you got, but this one looks decidedly tacky. Shiny leather, childish stitching, a loud, garish color—it's got "return me" written all over it. "I hope you like it because it cost a fortune," beams the giver, "It's a designer label. [Insert name of famous popstar] has one apparently…" Before your very eyes, the wallet transforms: the shine suddenly oozes hip street chic, childish becomes artistic, and what was going right back to the store, suddenly goes straight into your pocket. It's called perception: if we perceive something as expensive, it becomes valuable. Do your own designer branding by placing a value on your own worth: in other words, act like you're worth a billion and she'll see you that way as well. I'm not talking about pretending you're wealthy or acting like you're way out of her league; I'm talking about behaving as though you're well and truly worthy of her affection. Which you are. The trick to pulling it off? Be attentive but not 24/7 available; pay compliments but keep her guessing. That all sounds complicated, but it's very easy if you follow one simple rule: don't shut out the rest of your life, just because she's in it. That way, friends/work/life will naturally intrude on your time and you won't be there to return every phone call seconds after she's called or see her every time she clicks her fingers. The second bit of sneakery: pile on the"'I think you're great"

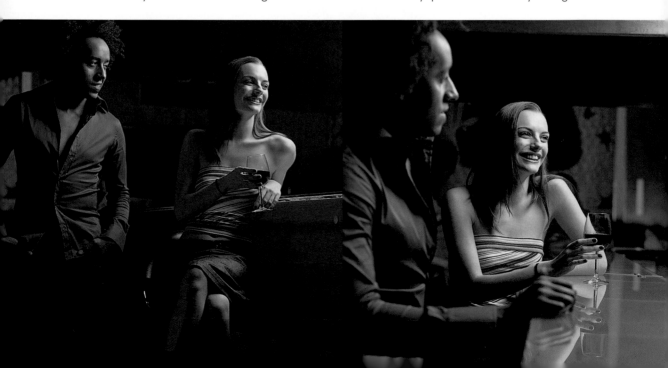

flattery without telling her how much you seriously like her. In other words, keep it as a general compliment ("You've got such a great smile"), rather than a protestation of love ("Every time you smile my heart flip-flops"). Later, she'll kill to hear it. Lay on the lines too fast, too thick, too early, and they'll all seem meaningless.

- **Track her down** Calling up to say, "How did that meeting go?" rather than the usual "How are you?" will put you light-years ahead of the competition. If you can't remember half the stuff she rattles on about, take notes. Seriously. Write things like "Ask if Sarah's sister had baby" and "S goes to doctor today" in your diary. Refer to it. If you're really eager this should come naturally but sometimes the opposite happens—you're so nervous about getting everything else right, you forget the obvious. It's called tracking, and it shows you've been listening and you care.

ON A ROLL

- **Avoid an argument** You've had a few great dates and now this! As far as you're concerned, it's crystal clear you're right and she's wrong. Sadly, she's behaving as though you're speaking in tongues (and not the kind she usually likes) and can't seem to get your point at all. If this happens to you, do something (anything) to get her moving. The quickest way to budge a mind lock is to get someone to change their body position. If she's sitting down, invent a reason for her to get up and walk around the room. If she's standing, get her to sit down. When our body is in a fixed position, our mind becomes frozen as well. There's no easier way to snap someone out of something than to get them to move.

- **Capture the moment** The opposite is also true. If you're locked together in a moment so intimate, you're afraid to breathe lest you ruin it, you're wise to grit your teeth and hang on (no matter how desperate the urge to pee). Get the timing wrong by "abandoning" he—lean back, leave to go to the bathroom, attract the attention of the waitress for another drink—and you may lose the opportunity to move the relationship onto a deeper, more intense level.

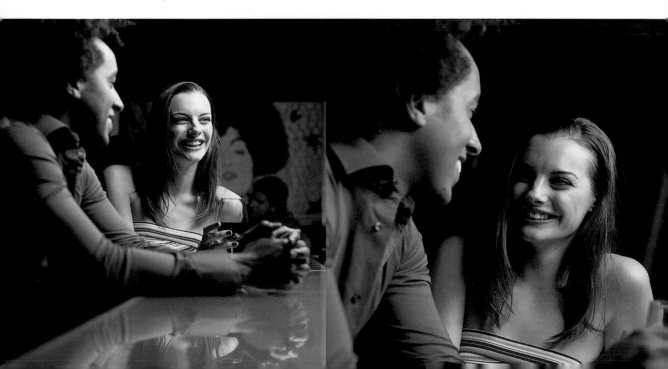

To take you places fast

Legs speak volumes about our true intentions and all of us find ourselves flirting with our feet. Decipher their deepest secrets and discover what's really going on by keeping your eye on the bottom line.

I have a friend who I'm incredibly attracted to, as is he to me. We confessed this after a billion bottles of wine one night, but for a billion boring and complicated reasons, neither of us is prepared to act. While our heads accept the logic, and mentally we've moved on, our bodies refuse point-blank to give up. Take the other night. We plonked ourselves in separate armchairs and settled in to watch a video, both facing forward in typical TV-watching mode. Totally engrossed, our bodies rearranged themselves without our permission. The credits rolled and we looked down to see ourselves practically climbing out of our seats toward each other. Arms dangled over the edge of our chairs, our bodies had turned away from the screen and toward each other, one leg stretched forward and our ankles intertwined. "Geez," we said, "And that's without a drink!"

We put on the face we want others to see but as we travel away from it, our body language starts to reveal our true feelings. Hands are halfway down and we're semi-aware that they're liable to "leak" secret emotions. Legs and feet, however, are completely forgotten and tend to be left to their own devices—which is why they're so remarkable for giving clues about what's really going on…

THEY'RE INTERESTED IF:
- **Their feet point toward you** If they're standing, one leg will move a step in your direction.
- **Their legs are crossed and the top leg points toward you** The direction of the leg cross is important. If you're sitting side by side and they cross toward you, you're on friendly turf.
- **They're sitting with legs wide apart and feet firmly planted on the floor, directly facing you** This person is confrontational, secure, sexual, and effectively saying, "Here I am. Take a good look at what's about to be yours." If they're leaning forward and fixing you with a steady gaze, there's good reason why you feel like a lamb before the slaughter. They're moving in for the kill.
- **Playing footsie** People tend to use this technique in situations where it would be embarrassing to be seen obviously flirting with someone. Like a group of work colleagues out for the night or at a friend's dinner party where everyone's married. It works like this: they put their foot next to yours so it's touching. You don't move. They snuggle their foot in closer so you know it's not a mistake; you apply slight pressure back. If they risk stroking your foot with their toes and you still don't budge or you reciprocate, it's the equivalent of saying, "I will go home with you".

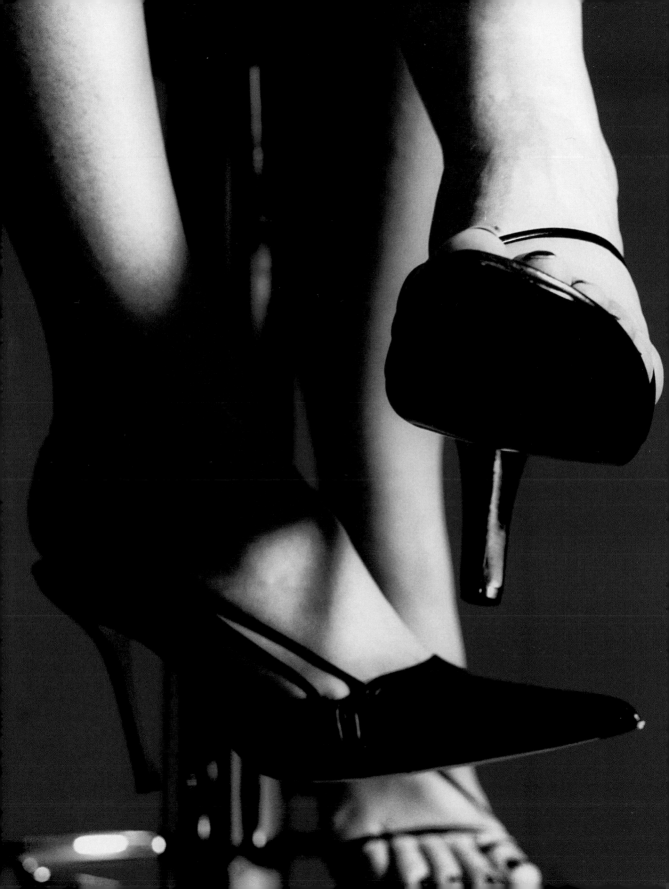

SHE'S INTERESTED IF:

As a guy, you get extra info because women use their legs to send more flirting signals than men. Why? Because, as I said, men's parts get in the way.

- **She's crossed her legs at the thighs** The classic "I'm interested" female flirting signal. So clichéd, it's potent—everyone can read it, and everyone responds to it.
- **The double twist** If she twines one leg around so her foot crosses behind her calf and also the ankle, you're even more in luck. Hinting at creativity (it's a little more imaginative than a normal leg cross), flexibility (always handy), and coiled springlike tension (if she's physically wound herself in a knot, it must mean pent up sexual frustration—which you, of course, will be happy to relieve.) Favored by tall women with gazelle-length limbs (it works better with long legs than short) this pose is often paired with a little girl gesture—like a finger, seductively twirling hair—to downplay any possible height superiority.
- **She keeps on crossing and uncrossing her legs** The more deliberately it's done, the more interested she is. It's a not-so-subtle ploy to draw attention to the legs and genital area.
- **She's kicking one leg up and down, while crossed, or dangling a shoe from her toes** This girl's up for more than just coffee. It's a thrusting motion designed to mimic more intimate thrusting. Gulp.
- **She slips her foot slightly out of her shoe** She's incredibly comfortable with you and the situation. It's the old "kick your shoes off and make yourself comfortable" thing. If you want to test her reaction, do it now. If she feels ill at ease, that shoe will be shoved back on very quickly.

NOT SO GREAT FOR EITHER SEX...

- **Their legs are crossed but your instinct tells you all is not well** The standard leg cross—right leg rested over left—is usually a sign that someone is relaxed but it can also be a subtle way of protecting and forming a barrier. This is where is all gets a bit tricky. There's crossing legs in a sexy way to say "Check them—and me—out" and there's crossing legs to say "Stop looking at them and me". After all, keeping the upper thighs pressed together hides our most vulnerable area—the crotch. Look elsewhere to figure which message applies. If they've folded their arms, turned their head away, and averted their eyes, it's not good news. If they've recently plopped a bag or briefcase or pillow on their lap, even worse. The ultimate "piss off," would be for them to lean forward and away from you, lifting a shoulder to form a third barrier in effect. (Don't even bother saying goodbye, just slink away.)
- **They do the opposite of what you do** If they seem intent on adopting a different leg than you, they're showing dominance or trying to emphasize how unlike you both are ("See? We even sit differently."). Not a particularly welcome sign if you're so eager you're practically panting.
- **Their legs are tightly crossed** The tighter the cross, the more defensive the mood. If you're chatting to a woman and she lifts one leg, bends it at the knee and wraps her hands around it, hugging it to her, back off. This is a classic protect-the-genitals position. Watch young girls forced to be nice to men they perceive to be "creepy" and they'll adopt this position involuntarily.

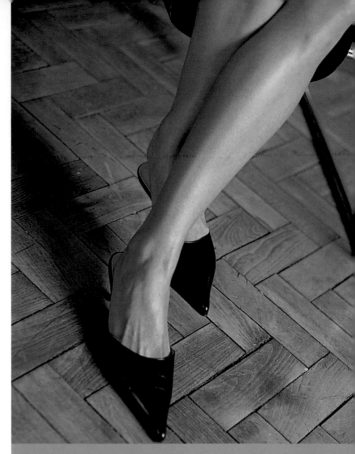

- **They're rising up and down on their heels, swaying from side to side (sober), tapping their feet, shifting weight from foot to foot, or doing any sort of leg or feet jiggling** All point to a secret desire to walk or run away. This could be prompted by fear (they like you but you frighten the hell out of them) or disinterest. They might pretend to be fascinated and/or totally at ease but their feet are trying every possible way to get them out of there by trying to run without moving. Ease up on the flirting, make general soothing chit-chat, and see if it stops. If it does, it's safe to assume they were nervous and/or feeling intimidated. Didn't work? Sorry, but it probably does mean you're not their cup of tea! Be graceful. Gather those few tatters of dignity you have left, wrap them around your shoulders, give a theatrical yawn, and tell them as much as you're enjoying yourself, you really must go home.

- **They've crossed their legs and one foot is flapping up and down** They're tense and anxious about where it's all going to lead or impatient for things to start. It's a "let's get this over with" or "let's get on with it" movement. Judge quickly and act immediately. If you're in heavy flirting mode, it's a female doing it to you, and it's a bigger, more noticeable, faster movement, this is a VERY GOOD SIGN. She's not just eager to move things along, she's impatient for things to progress NOW. Grab the moment or you might just lose it (and her). If all the other signs—sadly—hint at boredom rather than lust, they're trying to amuse themselves until you finally finish that l-o-n-g, story about the knee operation you had when you were 12. Sometimes the kicking is done so aggressively, it's as though they want to kick the person who is boring them. Given the topic matter, who could blame them?

Pick a personality from the way someone sits

- **Knees together, legs side by side, feet flat on the floor and neatly in line** The school goody two-shoes. On time, tidy, well-groomed, meticulous, not someone to throw around the bedroom. (Moving right along then…)

- **Knees together, toes together, heels apart** Shy and nervous. Coax out of their shell as you'd lure a timid kitten down from a tree.

- **Legs crossed at the knees, top leg slightly kicking up and down** Cool, scheming, thoughtful, ambitious. I suspect they've got their eyes narrowed as they sweep them your way.

- **Legs stretched out, one foot resting on the other** The ultimate relaxed leg pose. They're at home, confident, and self-assured. Study the circumstances they're adopting the pose in, and you've got a strong clue of what makes them tick.

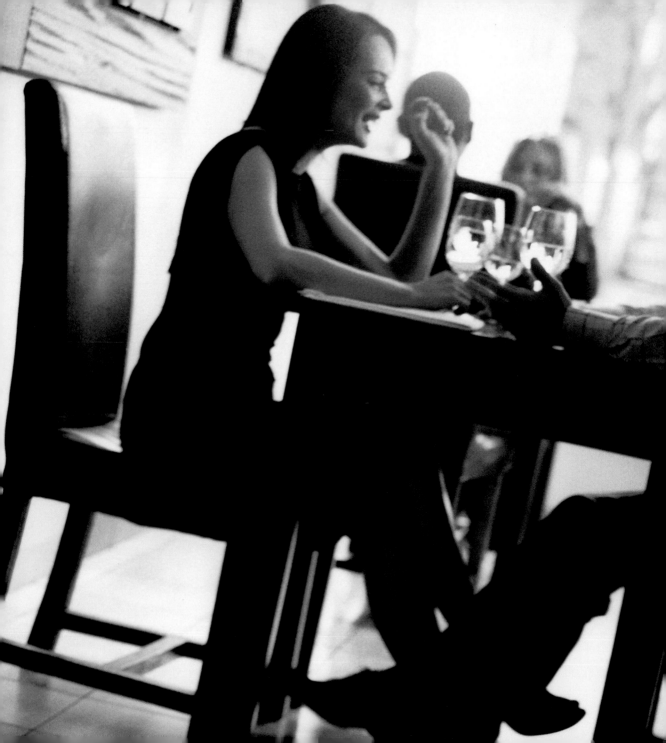

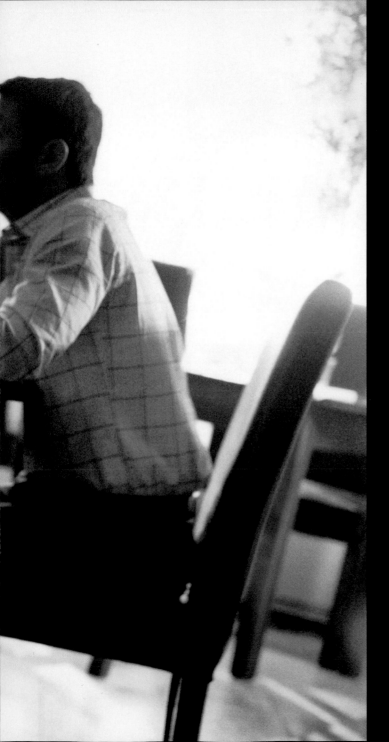

If you take just one thing from *superflirt*, make sure it's this. Mirroring body language is the single most effective flirting tool at your disposal. Forget model-perfect faces and bods, sports cars, expensive restaurants, diamonds, and designer wardrobes—in fact, all these can work against you! True friendship and love are usually possible only between people of roughly equal status. So unless you're both rolling in riches, one of you will feel uncomfortable. (I told you you'd like this book!) Even better news, mirroring—also called synchronizing or postural echoing—is so easy, you'd have to be a twit not to master it.

So how do you perform this magic? Simply match or imitate someone else's movements. Whatever they do, you do. Mirroring works because subconsciously we seek out versions of ourselves. Similarity breeds content—we like people who are like us. If someone is mirroring our behavior, we sense they're on the same level. We feel both accepted and flattered— which is why this one technique can turn a good flirt into a great one, instantly!

Sometimes, echoing is so obvious you can't help but spot it. Other times, it's the subtle gestures that give it away. Before you turn the page, check out the couple in the picture on the left. Can you spot the telltale signs?

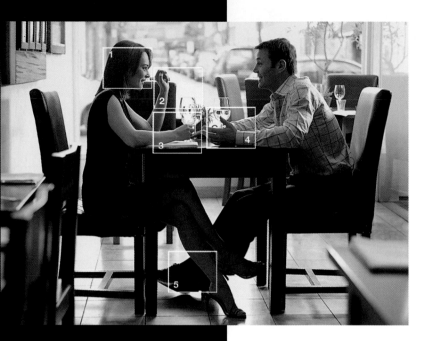

Mirroring ... **the**

Test them out

Check that you're on the same wavelength by seeing if they mirror your movements. Cross a leg, see if they follow. Wait a few minutes and try something else. If they don't automatically mimic the gesture, go back to mirroring them to increase rapport, then try again. If they're doing the opposite to mirroring and changing their position so you're racing to keep up, you're getting too intimate too fast. Back off— they're not ready to connect yet.

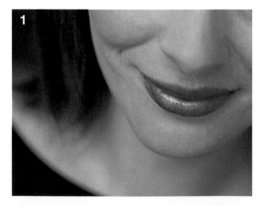

Verbal mirroring (1) Echo someone's head tilts, nods, and facial expression and you've already convinced them you hear what they're saying, even if you couldn't physically hear a single word. Match verbally on other levels and they can't help but adore you! Mimic the tone, volume, speed, and rhythm of their voice and you'll convey the right emotion.

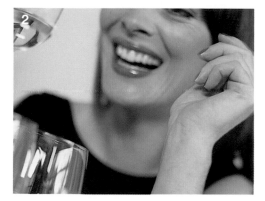

Exposed wrists (2) You don't have to form a mirror image of someone to mirror them: it's more about capturing the spirit of the position. While this couple's arms and hands are in different positions, the mood and message are identical. She's lifting an arm to expose her wrist, his hands are open, revealing both open palms and wrists. Both positions suggest honesty.

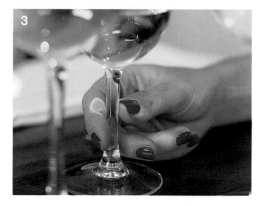

Fingers curled around glass (3) Both are holding on to their wine glasses: she's holding the stem, he's got a grip on the base. It's a great example of matching body language without "apeing." If you're too deliberate in mirroring someone, they'll think you're making fun. The ideal time to copy is between five and 50 seconds after they've changed position.

sincerest form of flattery

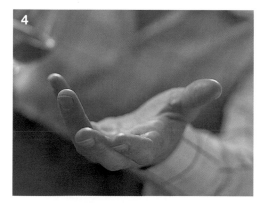

Outstretched arms (4) They "reach out" emotionally and physically, each comfortably invading the other's space. We mirror visually (body posture), verbally (the actual words chosen), and vocally (with our voice tone and speed). But the first one is crucial: 55 percent of us mirror with our body language, 38 percent vocally, but only 7 per cent verbally.

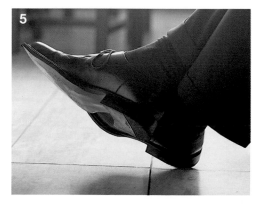

Confident ankles (5) Both leg positions mirror each other, half-reaching toward the other and a middle ground. If this were a moving picture, you'd be able to watch the couple do a courtship "dance." One leans forward, the other leans forward, she crosses her legs, he follows. The more synchronized the couple, the more attracted and bonded they are.

Is **he interested** in me?

Legend has it that men make the first move, then plead, cajole, wine, dine, and basically bribe (via chocolates, flowers, and dinner dates) women into their bachelor pads to either a) have their wicked way or b) get down on bended knee. Women—sweet, passive, delicate little flowers that we are—start out strong by defying his attentions, until sheer persistence breaks down our resistance and we agree to…a sherry. Meanwhile, we fill our days by reading romance novels and peering from behing the closed curtains, on the watch for knights on big white stallions.

What a load of crap. Women have always made the first move and orchestrated the pace, flow, and direction of romantic relationships. Masters of intuition and emotional manipulation, adept at body language, able to gauge the emotional temperature of a room quicker than our nipples stiffen in a breeze, you can bet on it that if he's on his way over, armed with courage and a pickup line, you were the one who lured him.

A **slightly surprised,** quizzical expression means he finds you fascinating. Or **completely nuts.**

Women choose from no less than 52 moves to show men they're interested. The average man chooses from a maximum of 10 to attract a female. Good news then, that the average female is usually very good at deciphering body language. Just in case you're not, I've included the obvious, along with signals that are more subtle, secretive, and (occasionally) downright loony. (P.S. Check out the all-important eye techniques on pp.42–45 for other crucial tips!)

IT'S ALL GOOD NEWS:
- **He'll serve you an eyebrow flash** When we first see someone we're attracted to, our eyebrows rise and fall. If they like us back, they raise their eyebrows. The whole thing lasts about a fifth of a second and it happens everywhere in the world—to everyone regardless of age, race, or class. Lifting our brows pulls the eyes open and allows more light to reflect off the surface, making them look bright, large, and inviting. A flash might be easy to miss but they're so reliable, if you do spot one, you may know someone likes you before they've even registered it themselves. Deliberately extend it for up to one second and you've drastically upped the chances of him getting the message you're interested.
- **His lips part** If he likes what he sees, his lips will automatically part for a moment when your eyes first lock.
- **His nostrils flare and his face generally "opens"** The raised brows, parted lips, flaring nostrils, and wide eyes give the whole face a friendly "open" expression.

- **He'll try to attact your attention** For some men, this might mean a subtle tie adjustment along with a silent prayer that you'll notice the flash of movement. Others turn into Bippo the Clown and become so loud and boisterous, they're practically juggling and doing handstands. Any exaggerated movement or gesture usually means he's trying to stand out from the group. Another giveaway: he'll unconsciously detach from his friends by standing slightly apart, hoping to be seen as an individual.

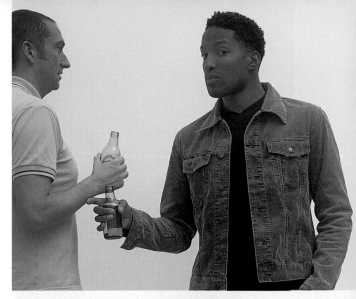

- **He'll stroke his tie or smooth a lapel** We all know what these preening gestures mean. They're the equivalent of the female lip lick— "I want to look good for you."

- **He'll smooth or mess up his hair** Which gesture he chooses depends on his hairstyle and what's going to make it look more flattering. Guys do this involuntarily and more often than you think. Glance back next time you trot off to the restroom and I bet his hands will be on their way to touching his hair.

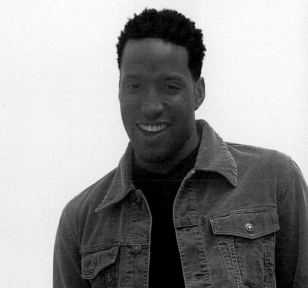

- **His eyebrows remain slightly raised while you're talking** A slightly surprised, quizzical expression means he finds you fascinating. Or completely nuts. Quite frankly, either are preferable to a man who looks at you with a smooth, relaxed brow and eyes. That one simply finds you boring.

- **He'll fiddle with his socks and pull them up** In the old days, men only dressed up on special occasions, and while the suit might have survived months in mothballs, the socks invariably continued to get worn (to death). Hence, why he spent half the night pulling them up, in an attempt to look the part. It's an extension of preening and it's astonishingly accurate. If a guy pulls up or adjusts his socks in your presence, it's an almost 100 percent sign he's interested and trying to look his best.

- **Everything is erect** Ahem. What I mean is he'll stand with all his muscles pulled tight, to show his body off to best advantage. He'll also stand directly in front of you to show full attention and lean forward to get closer.
- **He'll let you see him checking out your body** Some experts call it "visual voyaging"—his eyes take a little cruise around your body, stopping momentarily at the prettiest ports. Don't kid yourself: he scanned your body automatically the second he laid eyes on you. The difference here is that he's letting you see him do it. The message: I'm considering you as a sexual partner.
- **He'll spread his legs while sitting opposite, to give you a crotch display** He's letting you have a good look at what's on offer. Hopefully he still has his jeans or pants on at the time.

Secret **signals** he's up for it

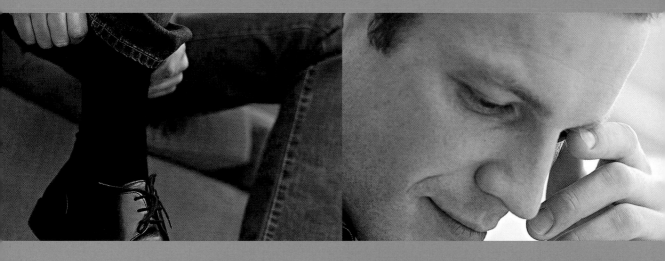

- **He'll stand with hands on hips** This accentuates his physical size and suggests body confidence. It's also a pointing gesture. We point with our hands at our own best sexual assets and also at the parts of our body we'd most like to be touched. If he spends the night with his hands on his hips, fingers splayed and pointing downward, he's willing you to look, touch, and admire the part he's proudest of. All subconscious, of course. Well, it is in most cases…
- **He'll move into "the cowpoke" stance** A variation on the above, the Texans named this gesture after researchers noticed men on the make—in this case cowboys—almost always adopted the same pose. Turned out it wasn't just Texans who stood like this: the cowpoke is a primary male courtship gesture of the Western world. He locks his thumbs in his belt or belt loops, points his fingers down toward his genitals, spread his legs about shoulder distance apart, and tilts his head to one side.
- **He'll play with the buttons on his jacket, buttoning and unbuttoning it** It's a displacement activity (fiddling) because you've made him a little nervous, plus an unconscious

desire to remove his clothes. The next stage is to push the jacket open and hold it there by putting his hands on his hips. If he takes it off completely, he's imagining his shoes under your bed.

- **He'll touch his face a lot, while looking at you** If he's interested, he'll stroke his cheek up and down with the back of his fingers, touch his ears, or rub his chin. It's a combination of nervous excitement, preening, and autoerotic touching. When we're attracted to someone, our skin (most noticeably our lips and mouth) become increasingly sensitive to touch and other stimulation. If you smoke, you'll take more drags on your cigarette. If you're drinking, you'll take more sips. You start touching your own mouth more because your lips are ultrasensitive and it feels good. Plus, it plants the idea in the other person's mind that it could be a good idea to kiss you…

- **He'll start squeezing his glass or can or roll it from side to side, slightly squeezing it as he does so** When men are sexually interested, they start playing with circular objects. Why? They remind him of your breasts: his body is "leaking" what's happening in his subconscious mind.

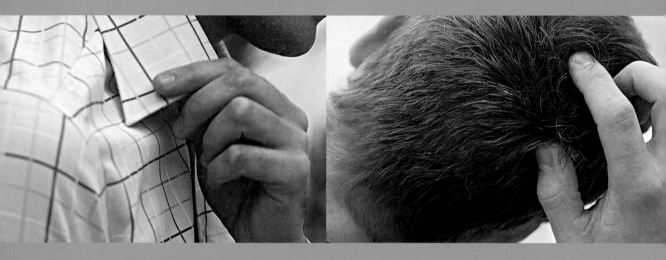

- **He'll perch on the edge of his seat to get closer** And if he crosses his legs, the top leg will point in your direction.

- **He'll guide you by putting his arm on your elbow or in the small of your back** The arm guide isn't just good manners and a polite way of guiding you through a crowd; he's making sure he knows exactly where you're going by taking you there. He doesn't want to lose you! It also shows you're being "taken care of" so no other men need volunteer. Along with the arm guide, there'll be lots of accidentally-on-purpose touches.

- **He'll lend you his coat or sweater** Few guys would be happy to return from the bar to find their girlfriend's evening dress covered by another guy's jacket. Never mind if her teeth were chattering from life-threatening hypothermia. He wants it to be his jacket because it's a protective, sexy, ownership gesture. It says "what's mine is yours," something that's been close to their skin is now close to yours (and vice versa when you give it back). It smelled of him to begin with; it'll smell of you when you return it. Plus, it links you: he has to hang around to get it back.

Is **she interested** in me?

Interpreting female body language isn't as difficult as you might think. It's firmly rooted in logic. Just about all flirtatious behavior aims to accomplish one of three things: get us noticed by the person we want, get us closer to them, and get them to have sex with us. (I thought you'd like the last one, even if the reason is procreation rather than recreation.) When we're attracted to someone, our subconscious goes on autopilot and gives in to a natural urge to get close to that person. Mother Nature, constantly snooping on our sexual urges, thinks "Here's a prospective population booster." and rings "all systems go!" alarm bells, instructing the rest of the body to look its best. She also connects with primitive mating urges, suggesting the body waft out some strong pheromone scents, and puts the body on sexual standby. (Is it any wonder we're all obsessed with sex?)

We stroke ourselves for two reasons: to draw attention to a **body part** and to **subconsciously tease** the person watching.

Understand the theory and you'll start to see that most body language gestures make perfect sense. (When I meet someone delicious—or simply feel a bit lustful—I start rubbing my lower tummy. Not only is this site fertility headquarters, but it also happens to be the place most females first register a pang of desire.)

If you're an intelligent guy, you've probably already figured out that women initiate contact around two-thirds of the time. Rather than going up and chatting however, they do it by giving you the green light to approach them, via nonverbal flirting signals. This is the sole reason why most men think they've made the first move—they're usually the ones who swagger over to speak. While it might not be the first move, it is possibly the bravest. Crossing the floor isn't easy and few women risk it. Reduce your chances of face-to-face humiliation by becoming a master at reading the sexual signals that drew you there. These will give you a massive head start…

IT'S ALL GOOD NEWS:
- **She's looking at your mouth a lot** It starts with the flirting triangle and becomes more intense as the flirting heats up. The more infatuated she is, the more time she'll spend looking at your mouth while you're talking. If you've been doing a bit of autoerotic touching (pp.170–73), she's got the hint and is fixated on it, imagining what it would be like to have your mouth on hers. Lick your lips and see her focus shift to your tongue. Gosh! I wonder what she's thinking about now?

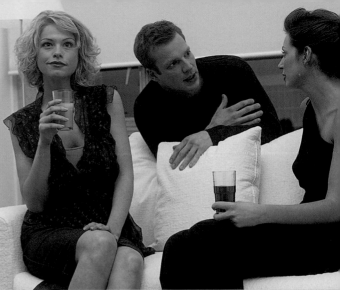

- **She's lightly stroking her outer thigh**
We stroke ourselves for two reasons: to draw attention to a body part (eyes tend to follow fingers) and subconsciously to tease the person watching (bet you wish you were doing this).

- **She's checking out your butt** Both sexes scan the body of a potential mate but do it very differently. Being more visual and usually more sexually aggressive, men scan from the ground up, eyes sliding over feet, legs, crotch, tummy, breasts, shoulders, and (finally) the face. Women scan less obviously and in a different order. They start at the face, having a good look at the eyes and mouth, then move on to hair and overall size and build. His clothes and accessories (a wedding ring, watch, shoes) are next, finishing on his legs and then back up to check out his crotch and…his butt. It's a long journey from your eyes to your ass, and the fact that she's got that far means you probably passed on the other counts. If you've been chatting for a while, glance backward next time you leave her to get drinks. If her eyes zoom downward, she thinks you're sexy. (If she's looking horrified, all those pizzas in front of the TV have taken their toll).

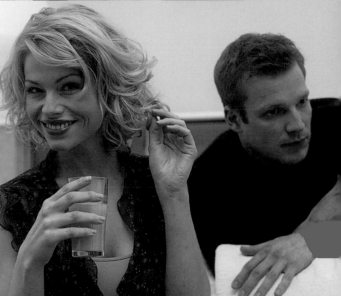

- **Her shoulders flash** When we meet someone we like we don't just flash our eyebrows for a split second (p.86), we also do a shoulder flash. Without realizing it, we'll shrug our shoulders when we meet someone we find attractive. It's a small, quick movement but stay alert to it if you want to be one step ahead of the game.

- **She lets a strap fall off a shoulder**
Revealing a shoulder is incredibly provocative. So is a glance back over one or stroking her own. Even shrugging your shoulders can be sexy if it's done in the right way.

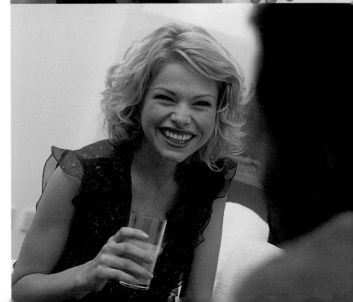

- **She starts massaging her neck** Didn't I tell you women are great at this manipulation stuff? She doesn't really have a stiff neck, she's just aware this pose lifts her breasts and exposes her armpit (another sexual hotspot).
- **She'll stand with her legs apart, weight on one foot and hips tilted** This is the stance of a high achiever: researchers studied executives at seminars and found 75 percent assumed this position within half an hour. It's also the posture of a sexually supremely confident woman and the equivalent of the male "cowpoke" (see p.88).
- **She'll dart short, repetitive glances your way** This says "Of all the things I could look at, you're the most interesting to me."

Girlie **giveaway** signs

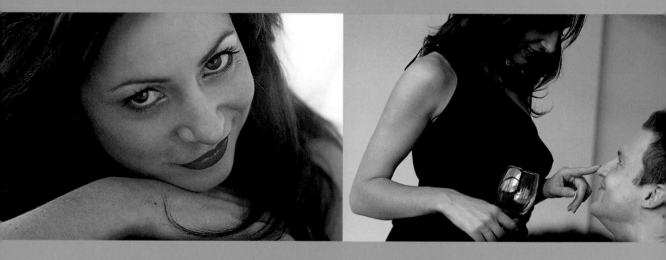

- **She looks straight at you and flips or tosses her hair** Some women toss, flicking their hair back with a head movement; others flick it back, using their hand. The second isn't just preening: by lifting her arm and brushing it through her hair, she's wafting pheromones in your direction from the sweat glands of her underarm (I know, far too much information). If she catches your attention, does either a toss or a flick, then looks back again, get yourself over there.
- **She'll flash her wrists** Wrists are a definite erogenous zone. Back in the days when women wore neck to knee clothing, the wrist and ankles were the only flesh ever exposed in public. Watch groups of women smoking to see a dramatic illustration of wrist turning as a flirting tool. Surrounded by just her girlfriends, each girl will usually have her wrist turned to face her own body whenever she lifts her cigarette to her mouth. The second a gorgeous guy appears, all wrists, magically and in unison, tend to turn outward or to the side.
- **She'll lick her lips, fluff her hair, and generally preen while looking at you** "I'm making myself look even more attractive—and it's all for you."

- **Her hands start to glide over her arms and neck** Yep—it's autoerotic touching at work again. (See pp.170–73 to find out what all the fuss is about.)
- **She'll do a whisper and lean** If she lowers her voice and moves her head close to yours, she's inviting you to share her personal space. It's a thinly disguised ploy—if she speaks so quietly, you're almost obliged to lean forward—but it works every time.
- **She moves her head closer to yours generally** The more we desire someone, the closer our heads get. The effect is two-fold: it excludes anything else from our field of vision and unconsciously prepares us for the first kiss. The most intimate prekiss position possible is where both your eyes are in line with each other's but still clearly in focus.
- **She'll sit with her inner thigh exposed** If one leg's tucked under her, revealing her inner thigh, and her head and body also point toward you, consider yourself wanted. She's revealing quite an intimate part of her body, one you'd normally only see during sex.

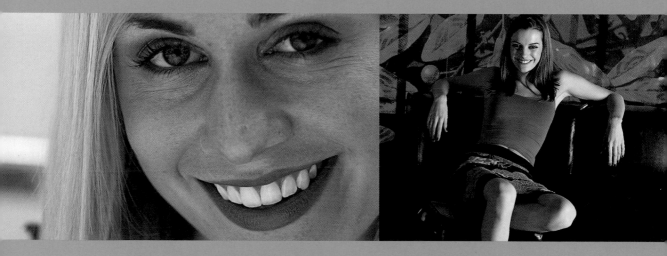

- **She smiles broadly** A huge, genuine smile delivered with direct eye contact is still the clearest signal of all she wants you to come over and talk to her.
- **She'll fidget with her clothes** When we're aroused by someone, our clothes seem suddenly restrictive. Lots of people start removing layers, undo buttons, or hike up skirts. Note how many buttons she's got undone and see if a few more have magically freed themselves while you were getting drinks. Keep an eye on her thighs as well (I know, it's a hard job) to see if her hemline has risen along with your expectations.
- **She'll start invading your space with objects** Unfortunately, it's more likely to be a wine glass, rather than the keys to her apartment or personal body parts. If you're in a restaurant or bar, she'll gradually push her wine glass from her side of the table over to yours. If she's confident you're attracted to her, she'll leave it (and her hands) there, hoping you'll touch them. Both sexes use their hands to signal interest by moving them into the other person's personal space, and stroking or caressing any object when close to you usually means they fancy you.

Armed and dangerous!

Forget childhood monsters and the bullies in the playground, it's potential or existing lovers, our boss, friends, and family who are truly frightening! Whether we're guarding against criticism or protecting our hearts from possible pain, everyone forms a protective barrier in some situations. Some barriers are physical. We'll hold a book against our chest, hug a pillow, or plop our bag or briefcase in our lap. Cornered by a sleazebag/the party bore, we'll hold our glass of wine or beer in front of us, positioned deliberately high, in a subliminal "piss off." Other times we use our own body parts to block or protect: most particularly, our arms. The most common barrier of all also happens to be the most well-known body language position: folding our arms across our chest. And before you jump in with a (defensive) "It's comfortable, that's all!," let me agree with you. My brother-in-law constantly folds his arms, but I know him well enough to understand he does it when he's completely relaxed. I also know he does it when he's angry. While some people do in fact cross their arms for comfort, just about all of us adopt this position when we feel defensive, protective, angry, threatened, or plain scared. Judged alone, as a single gesture, crossed arms might mean nothing. But if the person crossing them is also frowning, with a stony expression, narrowed eyes and lips pressed into a thin, tight line, I'll bet next year's pay check they are NOT happy.

BARRIERS

- **The standard arm-cross** Arms folded across the chest with at least one set of fingers on show. The tighter they're crossed, the more annoyed/defensive the person is. If the fingers disappear, you're in trouble.
  Fix it: Whether you're about to ask for a date or simply making chit-chat to find out if you want one, you'll get nowhere while their arms are in this position. Trick them into uncrossing them by handing them a drink, a pen—anything—so they have to let go. Alternatively, you cross your arms and mirror them, making them feel as calm and comfortable as possible. If you've done your job well, they'll uncross their arms the minute you do yours, following your lead.
- **The reinforced arm-cross** Both arms crossed over the chest with fists clenched and shoved beneath each arm. (What did you say or do to deserve this one?) Hostile, negative, about to enter the red-alert anger zone—if you can't fix it, get out of there!
  Fix it: Back off, change tactics, and generally beat a hasty retreat verbally, physically, and emotionally. Take a step back to give them space and so that they can see your face and body clearly. Stand submissively and apologetically—make direct eye contact, talk with palms up, soften your facial features—and change the topic until they appear to have calmed down. When that happens, slip in a subtle compliment or something positive about the situation. Once they've (literally) loosened up, that's the time to gently say: "Look, I seem to have upset you earlier. Please let me apologize if I have done and explain what I really meant."
- **The gripped arm-cross** Both arms crossed over the chest with both hands tightly gripping the upper arms. By holding on, any attempt by another person to physically unfold the arms

and expose the body will be foiled. Check out the knuckles. If they're turning white, they're really feeling tense. No prizes for guessing this person's not exactly overcome with confidence and the joys of life.

Fix it: By backing off and calming them down (using the techniques above) then trying a different way of connecting. The method of communication you're using isn't working. Work out if they're a visual, auditory, or kinesthetic person (see pp.58–61) and adjust accordingly.

- **The mixed-message arm-cross** Arms folded but thumbs are protruding and pointing upward. The arm-cross says "I'm being protective," exposed thumbs pointing upward says "I'm confident." Someone who wants to appear completely in control, even though they aren't.

  Fix it: Go along with the pretense that all is fine, but bolster their confidence as much as possible. Try to figure out what might be making them nervous and reassure without giving the game away.

- **The partial arm-cross** One arm across the body, touching the other which remains loose. This person's a little shy and anxious but not ridiculously so. Or they're acutely aware of the message that tightly crossed arms send, but can't quite help doing a half-cross anyway.

  Fix it: As above: don't go overboard with making a fuss but do pay attention and give them time to settle in and settle down.

- **The secret arm-cross** An arm swings across the body in an instinctive urge to form an arm barrier, but not wanting to appear nervous by letting it stay there, we do something—touch a bracelet, adjust a shirt cuff, or simply scratch ourselves—before dropping it back again.

  Fix it: No fixing required—they're confident enough to do it themselves, despite the (cute) flash of vulnerability unintentionally given.

While some people do in fact **cross their arms for comfort**, just about all of us adopt this position **when we feel defensive**, protective, angry, threatened, or **plain scared**. If the person crossing them is also **frowning, with a stony expression,** I'll bet **next year's pay check** they are NOT happy.

Tools of the trade

Straws, glasses, and other great flirting props

Sucking on the end of your sunglasses, teasingly twirling a straw, moving your fingers up and down the stem of a wine glass…Caressing objects is a seemingly innocent, but oh-so-sly way to let someone know you're attracted—without putting yourself on the line.

A cautionary tale for anyone planning on using a flirting prop: the nature of the beast means that it has the potential to go horribly, embarrassingly wrong. Brace yourself Mom, because I'm about to tell the story of you and the straw.

Emerging from a deeply traumatic divorce from my dad, my mother had (finally) picked herself up, poured herself into a (tasteful) little black dress, and headed for the nearest singles club in a determined effort to restore her self-esteem. A courageous enough move for anyone who's been married for what seems like a billion years, but particularly so back when "gay divorcee" meant a loose woman out to steal your husband, not a husband who's left you after stealing someone else's. Twenty-five years ago in Australia, the most hip-and-happening singles' hangouts were Parents Without Partners (Tuesdays 6-8 pm at the local school gym; no alcohol) or The German Club (Fridays and Saturdays, 8 pm till late; open bar). Sensibly deciding she might need a sherry or two to muster some Dutch courage, Mom gathered up her two best friends and found herself…pleasantly surprised. She's damn pretty, my mom, but there's nothing like a kick-in-the-teeth from a spouse to remove that ring of confidence. Drowned in male attention, it all went to her head. "Anyway darling," she told me later that night, clearly buoyed by the experience. (I, on the other hand, was haggard and had circles under my eyes from waiting up for her.) "There I was, swirling my straw around a cocktail the nice man at the next table had bought for me, when another man gave me the eye." "Oh," I said, coming to terms with homebody Mom transforming into Vamp Mom. "And I thought he was pretty hot as well (Hot? Where did she get that?) so I thought I'd flirt back." (Please God, don't let her launch into makeout details.). "The idea was," she said drily, "I'd fix him with 'a look' and then lean down and sip my cocktail through the straw, while looking at him through lowered lashes." (Mom as Flirt Queen— Could I cope?) "Except, instead of the straw going in my mouth, it went up my nose. In fact, it went so far up my nose, it pierced my brain! I tried to look cool—really—but it hurt, and my eyes started watering and then I laughed so much, stuff started coming out my nose and…oh God," she said, wiping her streaming eyes. "I'm not cut out for this. What a nightmare". When I stopped laughing, I said, "Never mind Mom, there'll be other men." "Oh I know that sweetie…but you never know, this one might turn out to be all right. After all, at least he's got enought of a sense of humor to ask

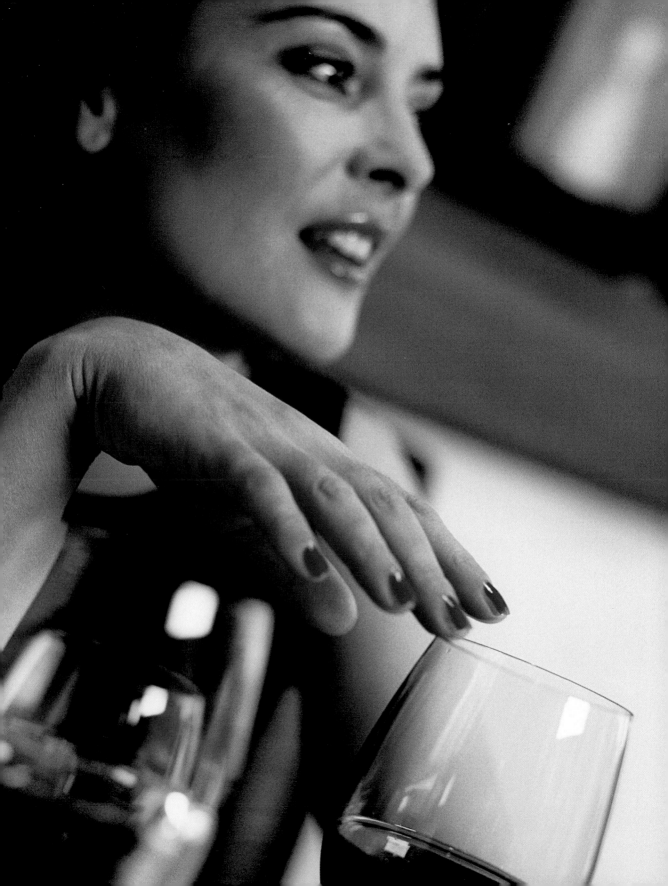

me out after all that." Moral one: you're never too old to learn from your parents. Moral two: perfection is someone attractive who turns out to be human.

THROUGH THE LOOKING GLASS

The trend toward contact lenses and laser eye surgery may eventually see the death of one of our most versatile flirting props—a pair of glasses. But never fear, the universe itself guarantees the next best thing—sunglasses—will survive, simply because we need to be shielded from the elements. And perhaps each other. Covering our eyes with opaque lenses has almost the same effect

> Putting any **object against our lips** harkens back to the secure feeling provoked by a **nipple in our mouth**.

as covering our face with a mask: it makes us anonymous. Any celebrity worth their salt realizes that if their eyes are covered, so are their emotions. A great idea if you're trying to retain some privacy, not so great if you're trying to get picked up or become closer to someone. It's not just the pretentiousness factor that stops us from approaching or revealing anything remotely personal to someone unnecessarily wearing sunglasses. It's also because it's almost impossible to gauge a true reaction to our words or actions without seeing the eyes. Sunglasses and prescription glasses can be used to great effect. You want to convey sarcasm and an "oh really?" demeanour: bend your head

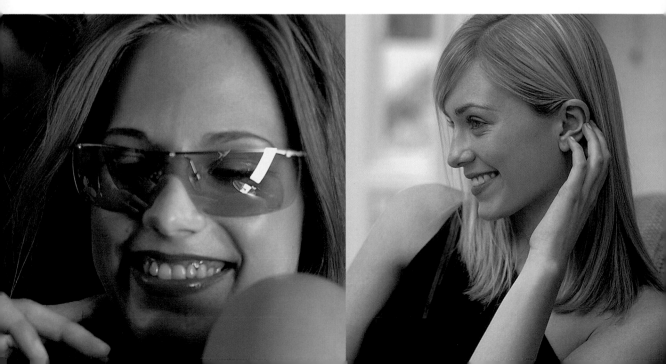

forward, let your glasses drop onto the bridge of your nose and peer over them. If you want to stall for time to gather your thoughts or let the person know you're seeing things clearly, take your glasses off, slowly and calmly clean them, then put them back on. Removing them decisively at a crucial, intimate moment means you're removing a barrier between you and that person and truly letting them in. Turn an emotional moment into a sexy one by following the total secretary-transforms-into-babe movie formula: remove glasses, let down and shake out your hair, then suck on the end of your glasses seductively. According to Desmond Morris, putting any object against our lips harkens back to the secure feeling provoked by a nipple in our mouth. (That's your mother's, not your girlfriend's.)

PLAY PEEKABOO

We do it as a baby, child, teenager, and adult: it's the "now you see me, now you don't" game. Mostly, it involves hiding then revealing the eyes. People play peekaboo using their hair, menus, other people, a strategically placed post, their hand, shoulder—virtually anything they can hide behind. We play peekaboo with clothes as well: jeans with rips in them, a top that reveals more when we lean over, a split in our skirt that reveals a length of leg when walking. Cute, sly, and playful, it's a body language move based on teasing—and an effective way to find out if someone's interested without putting yourself on the line too much. Looking over your shoulder at someone when you're walking or standing is flirty and fun ("I know you're watching and I'm interested, but you have to come to me"). Peering around something like a menu to catch someone's eye, then disappearing behind it the second your eyes lock, often starts an irresistible game. They'll keep staring to see if you emerge from behind it to sneak another peek and if they catch you, the combination of shyness and interest is endearing. If you're standing at the bar and spot a gorgeous stranger, it's much less daunting to flash a smile and then disappear by moving back so people obscure you. If they liked what they saw, they'll try to find you, or be desperately hoping you reveal yourself by leaning forward again.

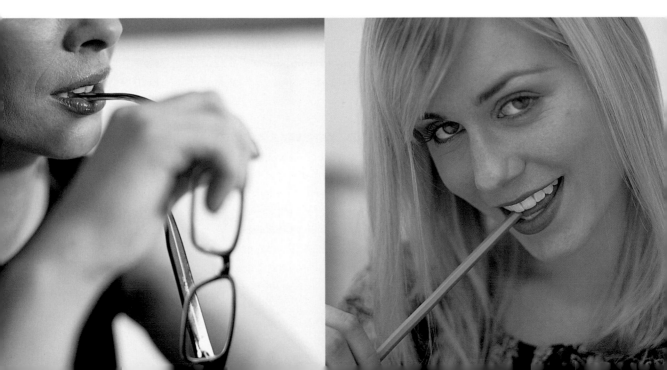

DRINK IN THEIR PERSONALITY

- **They're fiddling with their straw** It's a classic displacement activity—when people are nervous or bored, they unconsciously perform useless, repetitive actions. Most find it off-putting, simply because they're unsure of which emotion is prompting it. Even worse: twirling your straw while staring into the drink rather than at them. Instead, use the straw as a flirting prop: twirl it, dip it, or use it to trace around your lips, but whatever you do don't chew it! It looks unattractive and anxious and secretly hints at a subconscious need for nourishment.

- **She's caressing the stem of her wine glass or the neck of the wine bottle** Does it mean what you think it does? You betcha. The clichéd interpretation is usually right: our hands will often caress innocent looking objects in a way that suggests what we're really daydreaming about or subconsciously thinking. Women, particularly, start moving their fingers up and down cylindrical objects before stopping abruptly when they realize what they're doing.

Our hands will often **caress innocent looking** objects in a way that suggests what we're really **daydreaming about**.

- **They've ordered something nonalcoholic** If you don't drink at all, I'm deeply envious. Never having to wake up with that ohmigod-what-have-I-done? feeling would be bliss. Which is exactly why nondrinkers make drinkers feel extremely nervous. If you're a teetotaler, make it clear from the start and get the "Gosh, I'd better not have one then" conversation out of the way. Most nondrinkers I know are more than happy if their companion gets a little tipsy, finding the mood infectious. (If you don't want them to drink, best warn when you're making/accepting the date.) If you do drink, but just aren't planning to that night, be aware of the message it sends: "I plan to be good and not let myself go tonight". Quite frankly, many will interpret it as "I don't intend to have fun or relax." For the same reason the drink you order first often sets the tone for the entire date.

DOES MY OR THEIR CHOICE IN DRINK GIVE AWAY ANY CLUES?

Absolutely. Here's a quick rundown on the most obvious:

- **Long (often lethal) drinks that take the bartender time to prepare**—This means you're settling in for a while. It's a special occasion and the evening's worth making an effort for.
- **Cocktails**—A positive sign if she's ordered one; a trifle feminine if his has an umbrella in it. Ditto, sickly sweet premixed drinks packaged in girly bottles.
- **A massive mug or pitcher of beer**—Depending on the people and the venue, it can either appear deliciously earthy and unaffected, or common and greedy. I'd play it safe and order a normal size glass. Besides, it provides a nice break in the conversation when one of you

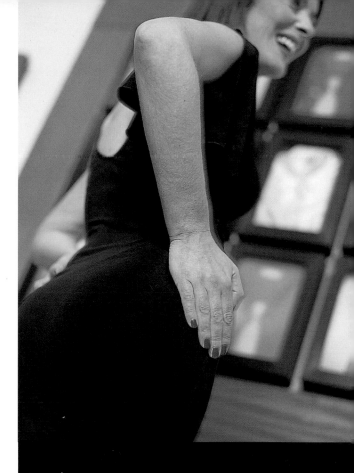

gets up to reorder. It's a chance to reflect on how it's all going, an excuse to touch as they hand your drink over, and a chance to share if you opt for a bottle.

- **Spirits minus mixers (on the rocks)**—A no-no for lots of reasons. No1: It brands you as a heavy drinker, working your way up to alcoholic. No 2: They'll assume you're nervous if you need a strong shot. No 3: It looks like you're in a hurry, since it takes about a second to drink. No 4: You'll be sloshed before you can say "Tell me about yourself."

- **Spirits plus mixers** —A standard choice that gives away little initially but lots as the night progresses, depending on quantity. A safe choice, but the best drink award still goes to…

- **Wine**—It's sophisticated and it's a good talking point. If you think they know a little about it, ask "Do you know much about wine? It's something I really do want to find out more about." and gives them a chance to show off. If you're a wine buff, it's your chance to shine. Sharing a bottle is a nice early bonding exercise and both saying "Yes!" when the waiter asks if you want another usually sends a clear signal: you're eager for the night to continue.

- **Should you drink beer out of a bottle or put it in the glass?** Etiquette wise, it's probably best in a glass but if it's a premium beer, there's something quite sexy about swilling it straight from the bottle. If you're female, this could make you look like "one of the guys." If the guy's traditional and you are at heart, avoid confusion by using a glass.

- **Should a woman buy a man a drink?** Yes. The only exception is if it's a first date and he asked you out. I would always offer to share any bills anyway but if he insists and seems to want to treat you, let him (without feeling any obligation, in any sense, on your part).

Looking over your shoulder while walking or standing says "I **know you're watching** and I'm interested, but **you have to come to me.**"

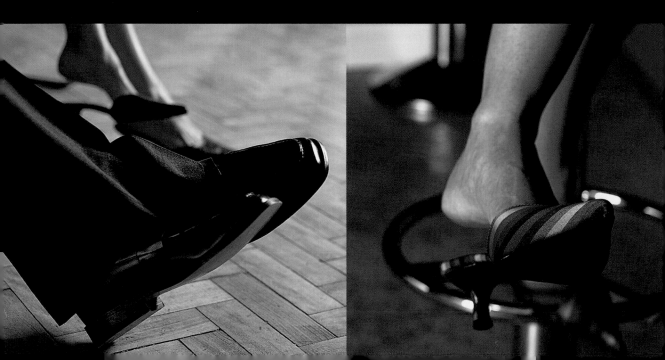

Playing **footsie**

Our feet are the most reliable indicators of our true feelings because it's the body part we're least conscious of and so least likely to control. Here we see examples of boredom (top left), feeling defensive (crossed ankles, top right), complete relaxation (legs spread out fully, bottom left), and seduction (foot slipped out of the shoe, bottom right). If a date goes as far as to remove her shoes (main picture), she's either too relaxed (i.e., isn't interested) or wants to move things along (i.e., get her shoes under your bed).

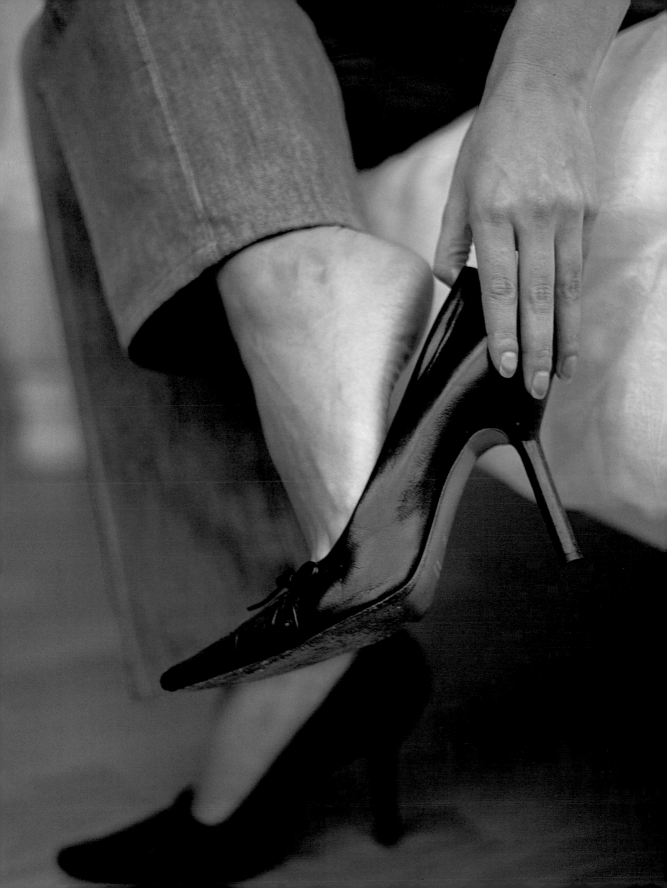

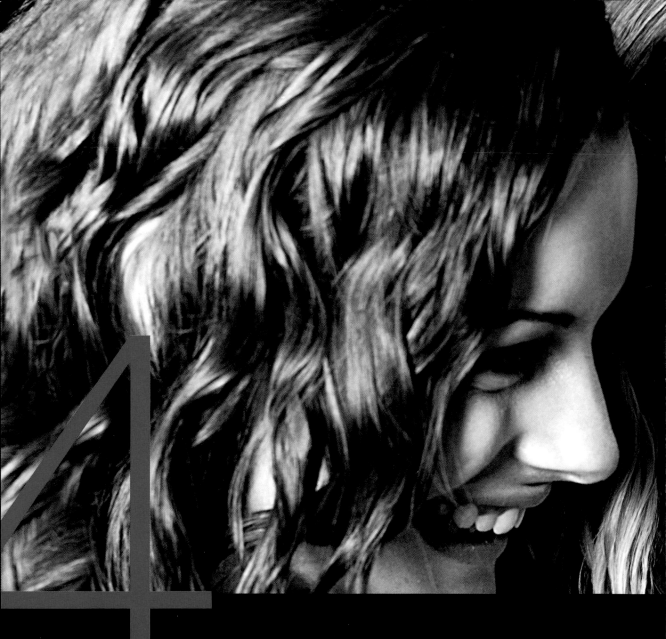

4

TALKING TRICKS

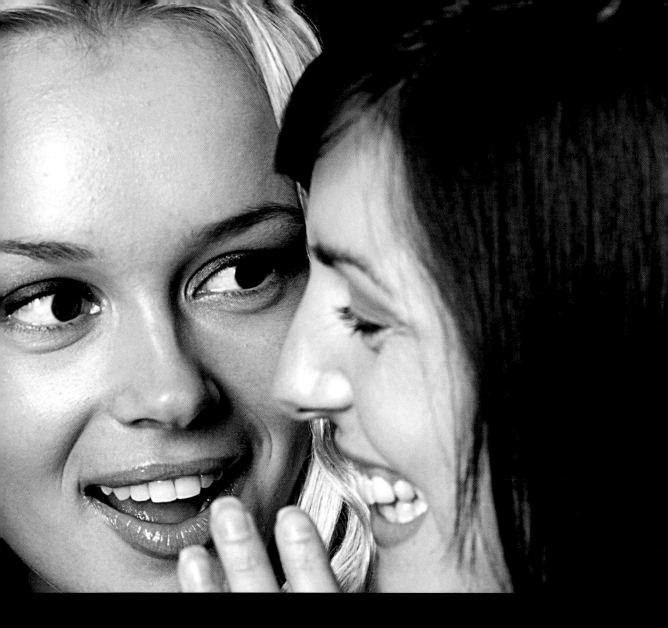

Back up body language with that other secret weapon: your tongue. How to talk so people listen, and how to listen so people talk. And, if all else fails, **read what's written all over their face.**

Sex up your sound
Time to start talking tactics

You smile tentatively, they grin back, and before you know it you're side by side. Do you a) Make Oscar Wilde seem like a bore b) Start rambling on through sheer terror c) Say nothing at all? Sad but true: the dishier they are, the more likely we are to answer b and c. Keep reading and start making sense.

If you've started at the beginning of *superflirt* and read this far, you'll have gotten the message that a lot of our communication has little to do with words. (The study of nonverbal speech—body language, voice tone, etc.—is called paralinguistics.) Experts say around 30 percent of our understanding comes from the sound of our voice, rather than what the voice is saying. This doesn't, however, mean you can run around ranting about absolutely nothing. Sometimes the actual words do matter, particularly in certain contexts. Saying,"Don't you have anything bigger?" to the grocer about to hand over a melon is acceptable. Saying the same thing to your naked boyfriend isn't.

Double meanings can also get you in trouble. A few months ago, I was at the supermarket when I ran into a girl from my gym. She snuck up behind me and said, "Good to see you've got a life outside the gym!" Which would normally be a perfectly acceptable thing to say—except that at the time I happened to have just picked up a rather large tube of lubricant. (Believe it or not—and I'm sure you won't—I was checking the spelling of the brand for my previous book, *supersex*.) I looked down at the personal lubricant in my hand and thought, "Is she referring to my sex life or the fact that I'm at the supermarket instead of on a treadmill?" Regardless, I'm now paranoid that she now eyes me suspiciously, no doubt convinced I am doing a man with a penis the size of an elephant. (On second thought, maybe it's envy.) Anyway, it just goes to show that the most harmless "Hello" can take on dark and dire connotations depending on the situation that you find yourself in, or what we happen to be thinking about at the time. And that's sort of my point.

This feature is packed with a plethora of practical tips designed to help turn you into a peppy, magnetic speaker and sought-after, sensitive listener. But at the end of the day, I'd still prefer it if you didn't stress too much about it all. We all mix up words from time to time, say the wrong thing, and go blank at the worst possible moments. The thing is, if you get your body language right, keep the mood light, and laugh it off, I'd be surprised if anyone even noticed! Keep that thought firmly planted in your brain as you practice all of the following, and you won't go too far wrong.

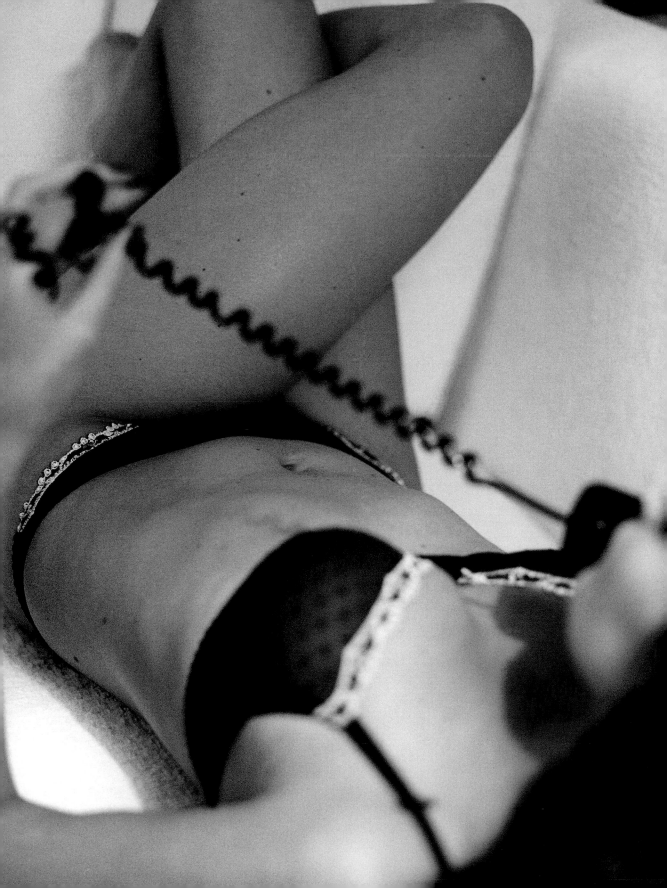

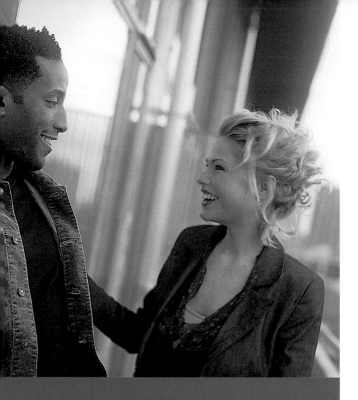

Instant bonders

- Use "we" as soon as you possibly can. "We're going to get fat if we eat all this, aren't we?" "Shall we have another drink?" Linking the two of you conversationally subliminally plants the idea of linking up in other ways.

- Another great word to use often: "you." Instead of "Anyway, I was talking about," say, "Anyway, as I was telling you." Including "you" makes people feel you're talking to them specifically and it pushes the pride button. It's also handy if you like talking about yourself. Include lots of phrases like "You would love it" and throw in the odd "Do you think I did the right thing?" and they'll let you prattle on for ages. What could have been a egotistic monologue is now an active discussion.

- If there's one word I don't want you to use often, it's "I." You won't just sound selfish if every sentence starts with it, but they might also think you're a bit nuts. One study found that inmates of mental health clinics say "I" and "me" 12 times more often than the average person!

THE KEYS TO COMMUNICATION:

Take a voice sample Match someone's mood and voice tone when you first speak to them and you'll bond much more quickly. Eavesdrop while they're talking, take a tone reading, and duplicate it. If possible, also listen for content. They're complaining about the heating? You'll make an instant friend by saying, "They really do need to think about the heating, don't they? It's a bit warmer over in that corner. Want to move there?" Not only do they feel you're on their side and sympathetic, but you've also instantly got something to talk about.

Mirror their voice Watch two close friends deep in conversation and listen to how their voices match in speed, tone, rhythm, and volume. The more similar your voices sound, the more the person you're speaking with will think you're on their wavelength (mainly because you are!)

Give good face Popular people tend to have animated faces and make a steady stream of expressions when they're talking or listening. Not only do facial expressions liven up our own stories, but they also let other people know the effect theirs are having on us. Evidence also suggests that by simply making facial expressions we can feel the emotion that usually accompanies them. Form a smile with your facial muscles and the brain recognizes the expression, thinks "I'm happy," and obediently releases the hormones that usually go with it—making us feel happier even if the smile was fake. (Smart little organ, that brain of ours!) If true, it's another reason to give good face: feigning enthusiasm could make us feel motivated; feigning sympathy could well help us empathize. Add to this the fact that a lot of expressions are infectious, and it really is a case of smile and the world smiles with you!

Be a parrot Verbal parroting is a great talk technique that gets you out of all kinds of ghastly situations. Basically, it involves repeating back key words or elements of what someone's been saying. This shows you've been listening and ensures that you've heard the right message. Not only does this guarantee that any misunderstandings are circumvented pronto, but do it continually and you can also keep someone talking for hours without any effort at all (giving you time to plot how to approach the gorgeous guy/girl standing in the corner.) Best to keep one ear open though, rather than go completely on automatic pilot. ("Hot in here isn't it?" "Yes. But I'm feeling the heat more than everyone else because I'm actually an alien and my home planet has subzero temperatures." "Subzero temperatures, eh? How cold are we talking?" Ooops.)

The brilliance of verbal parroting, however, lies in its ability to get us out of a tight spot. If you can't think of a thing to say, repeating back the last few words of what the speaker just said ("So you've known Sandra for two years?") encourages them to embellish their last statement, buying you time. Echoing

> **Trade secret for secret.** Make sure you start off small and extend **one intimacy carrot** rather than **the whole bunch**, complete with roots.

exact words or phrases someone else has used is yet another good bonding exercise. If they call movies "films," that's the word you use. Hearing their words come out of your mouth makes them think you share their attitudes.

Focus on feelings Focus on facts and you'll inform, focus on feelings and you'll also entertain. "How did you break your leg?" "In a car crash." Call me a psychic, but I suspect you're not exactly perched on the edge of your chair, waiting for details. How about this as an alternative answer? "Well, I was driving to work, horrendously late, and I was sitting in traffic, plotting what story I was going to tell my boss when all of a sudden, the car was moving forward and yet I wasn't driving. I looked in the rearview mirror and saw that a car had hit me from behind and was pushing me into oncoming traffic. The whole thing only took a few seconds, but it was so weird because I could see the driver's mouth behind me forming a perfect "O" and I knew I had my mouth open; and I could see this little yellow sportscar heading right for me and the sheer panic all over this woman's face, and then she opened her mouth as well. And all the while I'm thinking 'I know this is going to be a head-on crash.' And my last thought before impact was, 'I went through hell giving up smoking and it was all for nothing…' "

Not only is this story a damn sight more interesting, but it's also much more likely to get you some sympathy! Focus on feelings when asking questions as well. Instead of asking what happened next, ask how they felt when it happened or suggest emotions ("You must have been terrified!")

Don't make yourself your favorite topic of conversation The trick to people finding you interesting is that you find them interesting. We're all secretly fascinated by ourselves and the more time we spend talking about us, the better time we have. If you're trying to impress, shut up and let them get on with it. Nature gave us two ears and one mouth: use in the same proportion.

Open up when they do It's a bit of balancing act, really: tell someone too much, too soon, and you're wearing a badge that says "desperate and clingy"; leave it too late and you're "cold and hard to get to know." The trick is to disclose at the same rate as they're disclosing to you. Trade secret for secret. It doesn't matter who goes first, just make sure you start off small and extend one intimacy carrot at a time, rather than the whole bunch, complete with roots. Wait until they've shared something equally intimate before revealing anything further. Quite frankly, you shouldn't really be divulging the heavy stuff until you've passed through an intimacy sequence. Usually, we start by swapping clichés ("Awful weather we're having."), then facts ("I live in Chicago. Where do you live?"), then opinions ("So what do you think of the new mayor?"). Feelings follow ("I was really hurt when my father left us.") then it's time for the other stuff. If you're worried that you're spilling too much, too soon, check with a trusted friend before you blab. If your relationships fade before they've really got going, you've got the opposite problem: you're not telling people enough vulnerable stuff.

> # If you're trying to impress, **shut up** and let them **get on with it**. Nature gave us two ears and one mouth: use **in the same proportion**.

SEX UP YOUR SOUND
The right voice can heat up a room with a single sentence. A bad voice, like bad breath, can make sex appeal evaporate in an instant. Squeaky, strident, screechy, too loud, too quiet, mumbled, monotone—none will do you any favors. Give your voice supersex appeal by remembering to:

- **Breathe** Someone you're attracted to can "take your breath away" in a literal sense. When we're nervous or excited, often we stop breathing. Robbed of oxygen, your brain can't think clearly and your voice comes out high-pitched and strangled. Not the sexiest sound in the world. You might as well have written "You make me nervous" on your forehead. This, in turn, puts them on edge, and before you know it, the meeting's a disaster. Be conscious of your breathing when you're around someone attractive. Take relaxed, slow, deep breaths and you'll look and feel relaxed.

- **Match your voice to your image** If you've got a little girl voice, people assume you're girlie and giggly because, usually, voices match personalities. Hesitant, shy people tend to speak hesitantly and quietly; high-powered, people speak loudly and with conviction. Is your voice consistent with your personality and image? There's no point in repackaging everything else—attitude, body language, flirting technique—your voice also needs a revamp to reflect the new you.

- **Listen to yourself** Most of us get a horrible shock when we hear our voices on someone else's answering machine. Get an even better idea of how you sound by setting up a tape recorder and leaving it running the next time you have a friend over. Play it back and listen for different things. Do you make sense, talk coherently, give the other person a chance to speak? We all have pet words or phrases we overuse—what are yours? How's the tone and pitch of your voice? Are you flatlining—talking in a monotone? Are you speeding up and slowing down and introducing variety? Close your eyes and imagine you haven't met the person the voice belongs to. What do you think they'd look like? What personality would they have? Are they seductive?

- **Be a phone flirt** Because we're forced to rely on voice alone, phone calls can often go horribly wrong. Every word chosen takes on supersignificance when you can't see someone's expression as they're saying it. Silence is nearly always taken as disapproval. A rise in tone must mean they're angry. Not hearing any "go on" sounds must mean the person's not really listening. Often, we're right in our impressions. You can hear someone smile because their voice changes. You can hear if someone's offended because they'll stop breathing for a little while or start breathing very heavily. (And while we're on the topic of heavy breathing, you probably won't get away with doing that either!) The best way to avoid miscommunication during a telephone call is to imagine the person is in the room with you and adopt the same expression and body language. Chances are they'll "see" you through your voice.

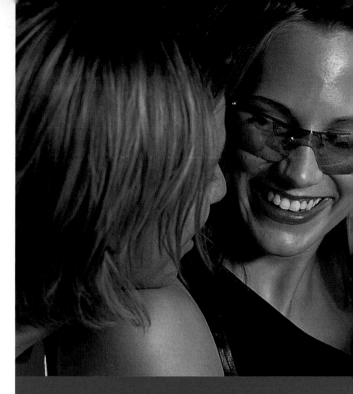

Instant intimacy

Create an instant shared past with someone you like and you'll create intimacy. It's easy to do: simply refer back to anything that's already happened between you. Say, for instance, you nearly spilled your glass of red wine on your clothes when the two of you were walking back from the bar. Later, the group conversation turns to white being the new fashion color for spring. "I don't think it'd be a good idea for me to wear white clothes, do you John?," you say, with a conspiratorial grin. The rest of the group is wondering "Why? What happened between those two?" It makes it look as though you've got a shared history when what really happened between you was inconsequential. Another swift route to instant attention: saying someone's name. Narcissistic creatures that we are, our name is the single sound all humans respond to the quickest. Try dropping their name into the conversation every five minutes and you will immediately gain their attention, leaving them much more vulnerable to your next flirting move.

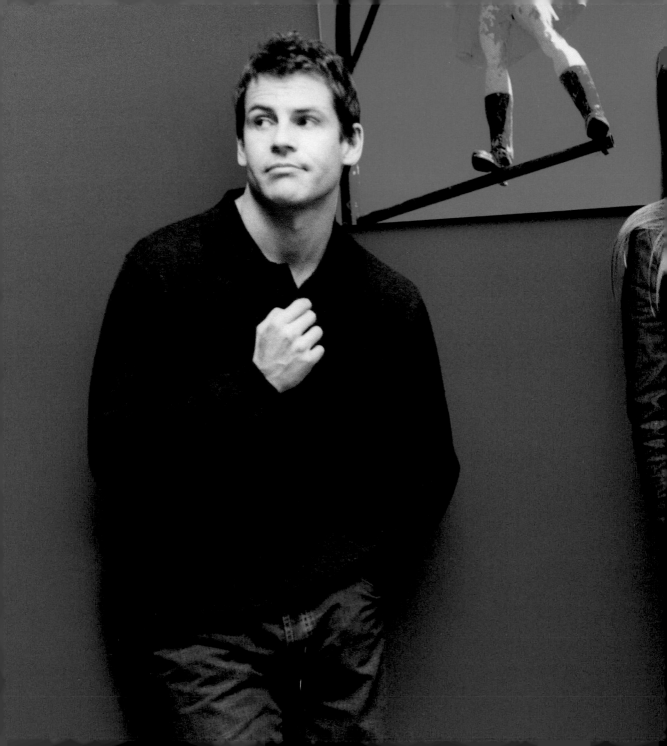

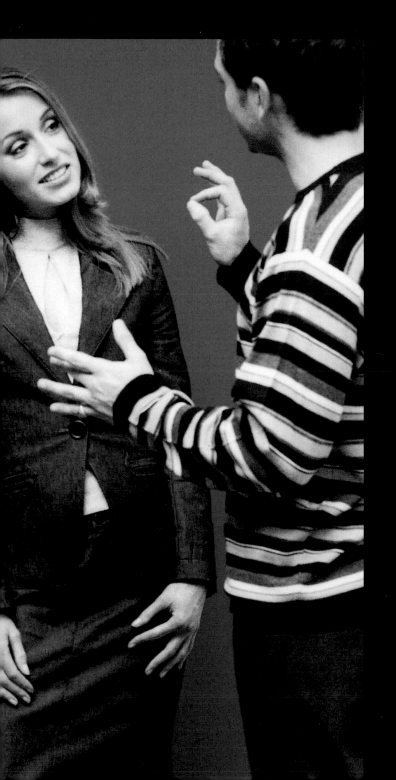

At the next party you go to, find the most popular speaker in the room (they'll be surrounded by a group of people). Stand close, but not so close you can hear, and simply observe. Bet you're equally entertained just watching. The people we find most fascinating to listen to often put on quite a performance, throwing their inhibitions away and their hair, hands, and torso all over the place to illustrate what they're saying. Watch carefully and you'll also see they're observing everyone else! Being a great talker means knowing when not to talk. If you spot someone on the brink of boredom, you can save the situation by swiftly switching topics or getting them to talk—before they've even noticed you were less than wonderful. Impress them by listening while someone else takes center stage. Lots of us think of listening as something to be endured before we can get back to the good part—talking. Which explains why the rare person who really listens is so relished: they're popped straight in the special basket. There's a difference between speaking and talking, and a difference between hearing and listening. It's in your interest to know what the difference is. The clues are all hidden in this picture. One glance will tell you who's bored and who's interested. That's the easy part. The secret is deciphering all the details that gave you this impression. Turn the page to find out.

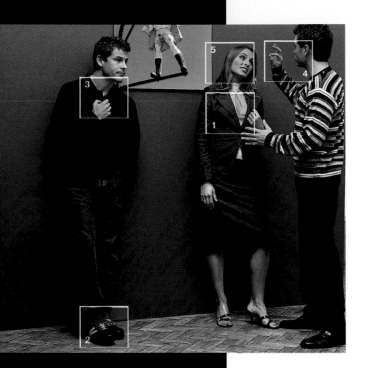

How to listen so

Listening tips

- We all have a habit of finishing people's sentences, assuming we know exactly what they were about to say. If it's someone you want to get to know better, let them say their piece.

- A nod is one of the simplest but most effective "keep going" gestures you can make. If someone's belaboring a point, talking too slowly or too much, nod faster and more often.

- The best listeners act as mirrors for the conversationalist, reflecting their emotions.

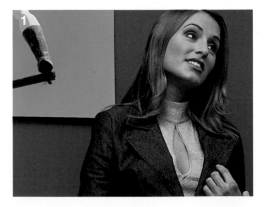

Be an active listener (1) Listen not just with your ears but your entire body. Show you're hearing them. Smile, frown, widen your eyes, lean forward, move to the edge of your seat, encourage verbally with lots of "uh huh's." If you're having trouble relating but want to show sympathy, copy their expressions, right down to the side-to-side and up-down head motions.

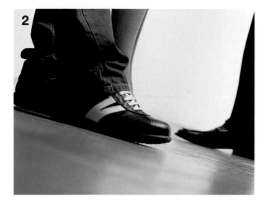

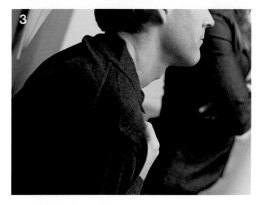

The intention movement (2) Another example of our body betraying our real feelings is the intention movement. This is a body poised to leave. His feet are positioned ready to walk straight out the door and his torso is turned toward the exit. Intention gestures are small, preparatory movements revealing what we're about to do.

Spot the slump (3) Our legs aren't the only things which give us away: our torso—quite literally—lets us down. Excited people stand or sit straight and tall. Boredom makes our entire body slump and sag until we're practically slipping down the wall or falling off our chair. The second you see people start to slide, change the subject or ask for their feedback.

people talk...

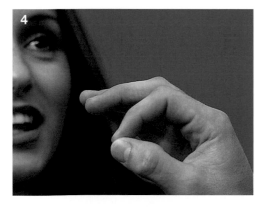

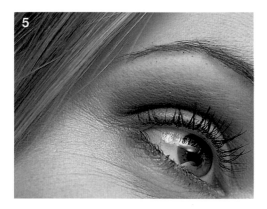

Pay attention to the fingers (4) We use the whole hand for a "power" grip (to pick up big objects) and join thumb and forefinger for a "precision" grip (to lift small or delicate things). When talking, we use each gesture in a similar way to emphasize particular points. We'll use a precision grip when we want to be precise: choosing our words delicately and carefully.

The giveaway (5) Is she really interested in what the man's saying? All the other signs say yes but the small pupils contradict it. You can fake lots of things, but you can't fake the signals your pupils send. If we're excited, happy, aroused, or feeling pleasure, our pupils expand. If we're unhappy or annoyed, they contract to pinpricks.

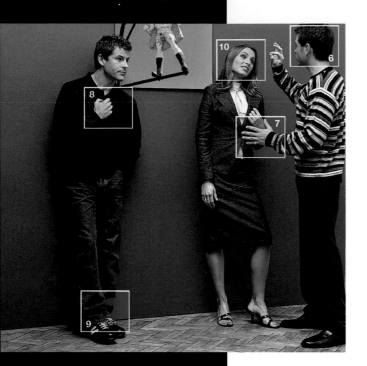

Keeping them

You were saying?

- **Women show interest by looking animated and throwing in lots of nods and smiles. Men do the opposite and show attention by remaining quite still.**

- **Listen don't plot! It's obvious if you're mentally planning your reply and not listening to what is being said. Your eyes drift away and become unfocused, and your brow furrows.**

- **We look at the person we're listening to 75 percent of the time, but when talking, only make direct eye contact 37 percent of the time.**

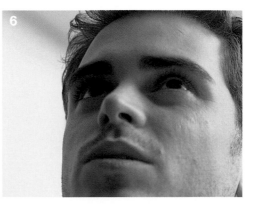

Look away (6) It seems rude, but it's normal to look away sometimes when you're talking. We usually start the story looking, then look away—to give full attention to what we're saying—then back once we've got past the hard part. Passionate people tend to look away and upward when explaining a difficult point, so we equate the gesture with interesting speakers.

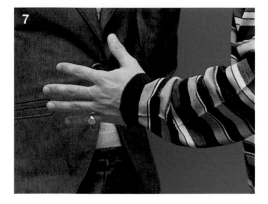

Draw pictures (7) Hands are excellent tools for expressing and explaining. This guy is literally drawing a picture in the air to show what he means. A good speaker's hands are seldom still, says Desmond Morris, instead they "flick, swish, and dip as he conducts the music of his words." Most of us are conductors, beating time to the rhythm of our own words.

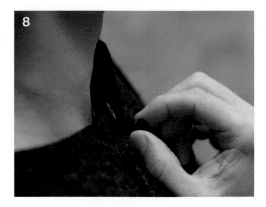

Focus on fidgets (8) Undoing and doing up buttons is a classic displacement activity—most people call it fidgeting. We make pointless and repetitive movements when we're stressed, nervous, bored, or frustrated. If you're talking and people are fiddling with hair, earrings, cuffs, shredding napkins, or stripping labels off bottles, then change topics, tone, and pace.

entertained

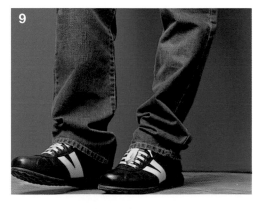

Check below the waist (9) Knees and legs jiggling and jumping, crossing our legs, and bouncing one foot up and down are all signs we're secretly longing to flee. Lots of us manage to keep our facial expression under control (we're very practiced at assuming an interested look), but our tense, restless shifts from leg to leg contradict it.

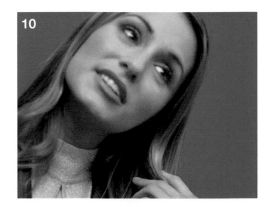

Tilt your head (10) If a woman tilts her head forward and to the side, then looks at you sideways, there's a good chance she's interested in you. If she pulls her hair away to expose her neck further, get her phone number. It's a great flirting pose. Tilting the head exposes the neck—an erotic area, rarely touched by people other than a lover.

The art of face reading

If you really want to know what someone's like, look at their face. Well, that's what Siang Mien devotees claim. The Chinese have been practicing the art of face reading for more than 3,000 years and say our features speak a secret language, telling all about our character and hidden desires. The Chinese proverb says, "The packaging is different, because the contents are different." No two people have identical faces, not even identical twins. That's because no one has identical personalities (thank God). The human face is capable of making 7,000 distinct expressions. We might only use a few hundred of these in everyday life, but those we use the most leave a mark on our faces. By the time we hit 50 you can determine whether we've spent most of our lives smiling or frowning. The astute can also pick up on more esoteric qualities with a glance, like who's been lonely or popular, a victim or survivor. If you've sailed through life, it stands to reason you're going to end up with a different face from someone who got stuck up the proverbial creek minus the paddle. Face reading is fascinating stuff, not to mention great dinner party trivia, even if some of it is varied and contradictory.

HOW DO YOU MEASURE UP?
Eyebrows
- Small and sparse: zero interest in sex; major interest in Zen. Think spiritual rather than sensual.
- Thick and bushy: sexually excessive. Feed with a steady diet of new erotic experiences.

Eyes
- Very pale eyes: Looking for new peaks and a quick fix. Easily sexually satisfied, they attach little importance to it or to love (not so good if you want a relationship). Changes partners faster than outfits.

- Dark eyes: passionate and into marathon deep and meaningfuls, hard to get to know initially, but you won't regret the effort. Dynamite in bed. Keep them there with lots of intense, varied sex.

Nose

- Snub nose: dreamy, into romantic sex and traditional positions—could translate to drippy for some. Not interested in erotic adventures.
- Bumpy nose: not a good match for the snub nosed, bumpy-nosed people are the complete opposite. Not only do they love sex, they like lots of it—the kinkier, the better!

Lines

- Small, thin lines under the lower eyelids: it's not something you usually look for…until now. This is the mark of someone with an enormous sexual appetite, who's constantly ready for sex. Nothing is forbidden and everything goes.
- Fine lines below the base of the nose: I shamefully own up to having these but insist it's from my years as a smoker. This is apparently a surefire sign of someone who rarely thinks about anything else but sex (Well, it is my job!). Blessed/cursed with the highest libido of all, they need to be loved in every way possible and are extremely hard to satisfy. (Not true. Honest!)

Lips and mouth:

- Large mouth: when it comes to mouths, the bigger, the better seems to apply. Large-mouthed lovers are unselfish and take time to pleasure. Men with large mouths are unbeatably potent lovers. If you've got a full bottom lip, score extra points—you're a sensual adventurer—minus points for also being shamelessly unfaithful. People with wide mouths are ambitious creatures who like to be the boss in the bedroom.
- Small mouth: imaginative and inventive, but that's where the compliments end. They're also quick to orgasm, wary of new people, loyal to few, and not very affectionate.

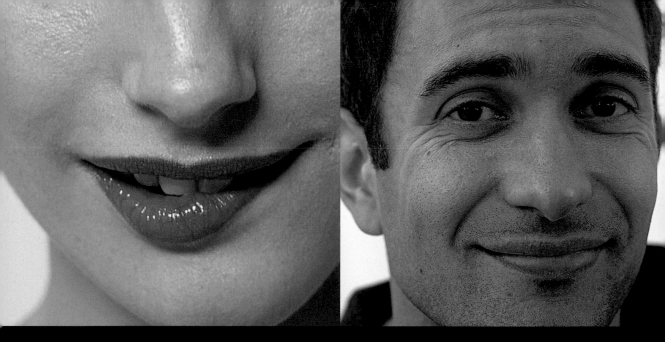

Mouth moves

The more we're attracted to someone, the more time we spend looking at their mouth. Although we use our mouths to speak, they also speak volumes without us saying a word. Here we see someone who's tempted but thinks he'd better not (top right), a fake smile (top left), autoerotic touching (bottom left), and a warm, genuine laugh (bottom right). Sticking fingers in your mouth while maintaining eye contact (main picture) is a definite come-on.

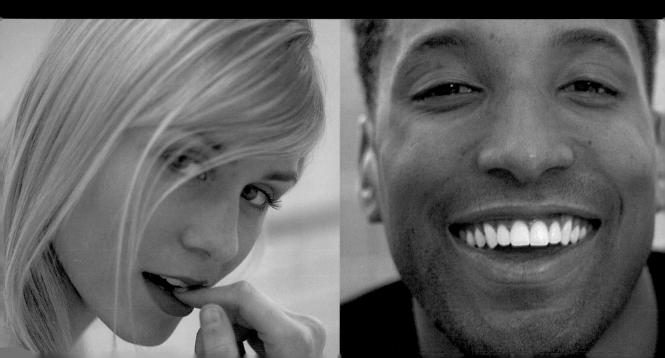

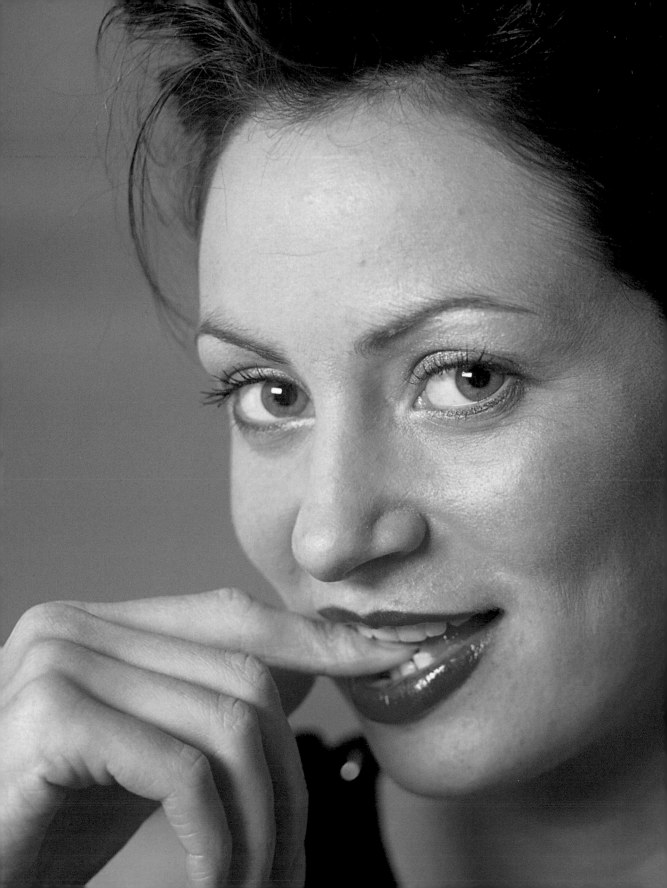

5

ALL-OUT FLIRTING

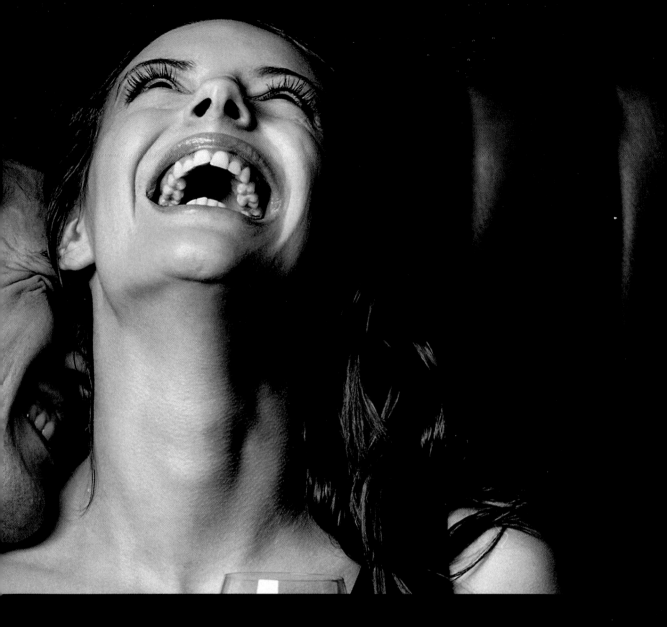

The really juicy parts: how to make anyone fall for you, touch them up, tell if they're flirting, or just being friendly – plus how to **pick up just about anywhere**.

The touch test
How well do you score?

If you want to connect with someone, there is no better way to do it than through touch. The briefest, tiniest touch can have an electric effect on how somebody feels about you. Lethal lust weapons at your fingertips—literally.

A while ago, my girlfriend and I went walking in the park. The fact that the park is enormous, it was subzero weather outside, neither of us have any sense of direction, and there was a heavy fog didn't deter us one bit. Within half an hour, we were hopelessly lost and thought it was hilariously funny. Two hours later, it wasn't quite the kneeslapper we'd thought. Suddenly, out of the fog, a black Labrador comes bounding toward us. A dog meant an owner, so we immediately bent down to greet and pat him, saying "Here boy!" A trifle desperately and a little too enthusiastically, as it turned out. The dog speeded up and as I bent down to pat him, jumped up to greet me—smacking me right in the face. Hard. Just in time to see what happened, a gorgeous man emerged from the mist. It was like something out of a romance novel. He rushed up and removed my hand from my cheekbone to "have a look at the damage" (I was holding it saying "ow, ow!" most becomingly. Not). Then he looked me in the eyes, cupped my face in his palm, and gently brushed his thumb across my cheekbone, asking, "Does this hurt?" Hurt? It hurt like hell—but, quite frankly, I'd have let a truck slam into me just to be on the end of that touch. Yes, he was sexy and he rescued us, but it was the touch that made the whole thing extraordinary. (Actually, "they" rescued us. Another figure appeared out of the mist—his wife. Damn.)

Absolutely nothing beats touch as an instant bonder—and if you don't believe me, try it for yourself. The next time you're out on the prowl and it's crowded, do the following experiment. Walk to the bathroom or to the bar to get a drink and gently move someone (preferably someone interesting) out of the way by touching them. Gently put a hand in the middle of their lower back and apply a little pressure to push them to one side. They'll look around immediately and when they do, flash the biggest smile you can summon and say, "Sorry! It's so crowded I couldn't get through." Assuming you've nudged rather than pushed (and haven't chosen the rudest person in the room), chances are they'll obediently move to one side and flash you a smile back. From that moment on, even if you're not really their type, every time you catch their eye, they'll smile at you. If you end up standing together by the bar, it'll seem the most natural thing in the world to strike up a conversation. In fact, it'd be rude not to because it feels like you know each other. All because of that one touch! Prove the point by repeating the experiment—minus the touching—by standing behind someone and asking them to move simply by raising your voice. Even if you do flash a supergrin when they turn around, the effect is

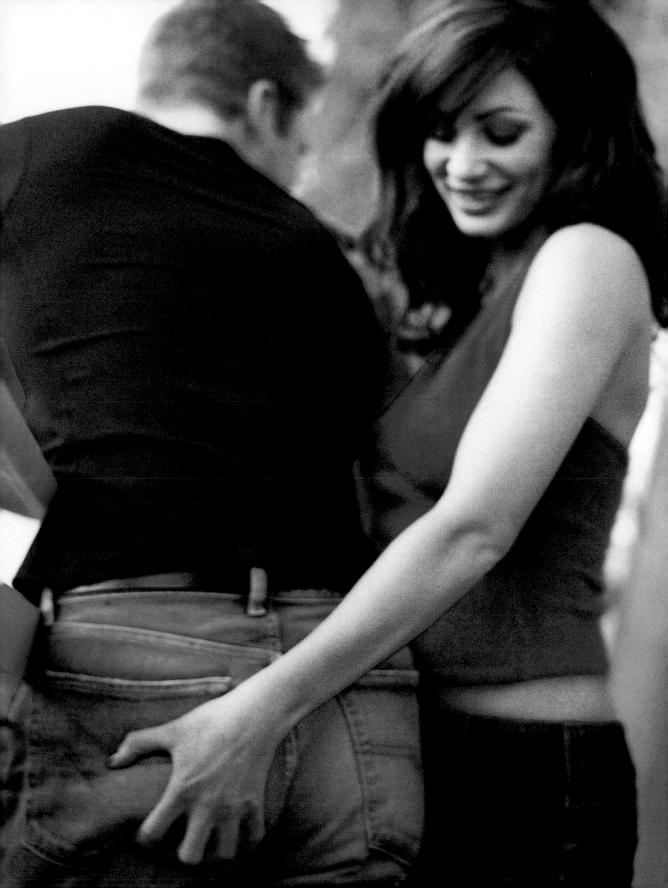

less intimate. They may or may not continue to make eye contact during the evening, depending on how attractive they thought you were. In the previous scenario, your attractiveness didn't count: you formed a bond anyway. Never, ever underestimate the power of touch. Fingertips are lethal weapons! The more you like someone, the more you touch them. Rather handily, the more you touch someone, the more they like you back. The first person to touch sends the first "I'm attracted to you" signal.

Being more interested in all this touchy-feely stuff, most women have figured this out by the time they're dating and will manipulate the situation to their advantage. Rather than appear too forward, women trick men into touching them, first by placing their hands or body deliberately in the way, so it's almost impossible not to touch them. If you keep accidentally bumping into her or your hands keep brushing, it's no accident. One of you is manipulating it because they're eager to kick-start the action!

> # **Women try to trick men** into touching them by placing their hands or **body in their way,** so it's almost **impossible not to touch** them.

Other ways to do it without relying on an accident? Point something out ("Gosh, look at that!") as you lean in to lay fingers on their forearm. Pass something (anything—a drink, a pen, the menu) and brush fingers. If you're the type who could carry it off, or you want to step things up to an intimate level, lean forward and gently wipe a hair from their face with your fingertips. If you want to be ultra-intimate, bring your face close to theirs as you do it. They might just choose that moment to kiss you!

According to American sexpert Barbara Keesling, when you're still in the flirting stage, you should touch for no more and no less than three times per meeting, each touch lasting around three seconds. The right time to instigate touches is in response to something the other person has done or said: if they make you laugh, say something to surprise or delight you, reveal something intimate, or make a point you particularly agree with, that's the time to touch them. At this point you're either feverishly taking notes or have given up, feeling it's all a tad forced and formulated. Don't worry. You do most of this stuff automatically. I'm just making you focus on it so you can use touch to your advantage. Absorb the messages, observe yourself and others for a little while, then forget about it, give in to your natural instincts, and all will be fine. In the meantime, you're still my student, so listen up!

- **The safest place to touch** is on the back of the hand, the forearm, upper arm, or shoulder.
- **Keep it gentle at first** Use your fingertips and skim, rather than press.
- **Time your touches** Suit the situation so it feels natural. If you want to hold her hand, wait until you're about to cross a street, then grab it—just don't let go once you've reached the other side.

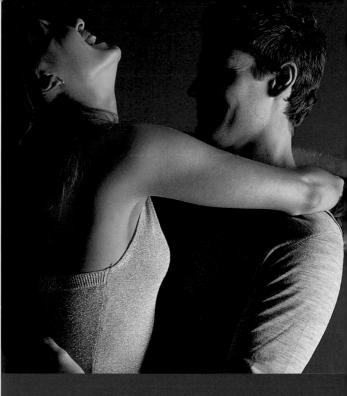

- **Test the waters** Use an "excuse" touch. They're nonthreatening, nonsexual attempts to (literally) make contact without putting ourselves on the line. If the person doesn't respond, it's easy to pretend you didn't mean them. Sit close enough so your arms touch, let your thigh casually press against theirs, move a foot so it's next to theirs. You initiate the touch, then let them decide how comfortable they feel with it. If they're interested, they'll find a reason to "excuse" touch back. If they don't, leave it. You've read the signals wrong: they might want to be your friend, but that's as far as it goes.

- **As you get more confident with each other** You'll find you touch more frequently (every opportunity you can get, quite frankly) and they'll reciprocate (every chance they get). You link arms, playfully "push" each other, happen suddenly to need cash from the machine at the same point just so you can line up together. You're not fooling the rest of the group or your friends, who are no doubt watching with amusement, but you are playing the game. And the game is important. It's what makes both of you feel comfortable enough to progress further. Given time, the touches start lasting longer, then become more deliberate and lingering, until eventually one of you takes a risk and makes a blatant move. Holding hands is usually the first definite sign you're both interested sexually and romantically. A kiss is final confirmation.

- **Certain touches will guarantee you a slap**, not a tickle, if delivered to the wrong person— or the right person at the wrong time. Each of us has a different sense of body privacy, dictated by our mood, past experience, culture and upbringing. As a general rule, body zones nearest to our naughty bits are the most taboo; those farthest away are the safest.

Hugs and cuddles

Close hugging in public is a dramatic "tie-sign" that indicates a strong personal bond. The tighter the grip, the more involved the person is (or wants to be). While lots of us hug hello and goodbye, only young or new lovers tend to hug constantly and face-to-face. Body language is highly symbolic, and by holding someone against your heart, so close they can hear your heartbeat, you're saying "I love you" with your entire body. Sexy hugs differ from romantic ones—the emphasis changes from lots of intense eye contact to lots of intense groin contact. If someone hugs you around the waist while pressing their lower body into yours, it's a pretty safe bet you're bonking, have bonked, or they very much want to in the future. The waist is close to our primary genital zone and only very close friends/family or lovers tend to hold us there. Most "public" hugs involve embracing the shoulders, not the waist. A waist hug takes things one stage further and women tend to pull away if it's done prematurely.

Make anyone fall in love with you
Scientific spells and potent potions

Some people will read this and think what I'm suggesting is wrong. I admit it's about manipulating and meddling with people's emotions. Most particularly, people you wish to God would meddle with you. In an ideal world, I'd agree. It would be preferable if everyone you wanted just fell in your lap, without having to play games. Unfortunately, real life doesn't always work that way.

Sometimes you can spend six months living, breathing, dripping, drooling, loving, and lusting after someone with zero result. And it's when that happens that the techniques which follow suddenly seem like a gift from heaven. Besides, it's not like I'm proposing black magic or suggesting any of these techniques will force someone to fall in love with you against their will. (If they did, I'd currently be shacked up with Brad Pitt.) What they will do though is nudge the odds a lot higher in your favor. Is that really so bad? I don't think so. Go on, keep reading. You know you want to…

HANG AROUND LOTS…BUT THEN BE UNAVAILABLE

The more you interact with someone, the more they'll like you, says David Lieberman, a US expert in human behavior. He's right actually. Several studies show repeated exposure to practically any stimulus makes us like it more (the only time it doesn't hold true is if our initial reaction to it is negative). So forget about being all aloof, evasive, and unavailable in the beginning. Instead, find lots of excuses to spend time with them.

Now, pay attention, because this is the tricky part. Just when you're convinced you've won them over and they like you, start being a little less available. And then even less, until they hardly see you at all. You've now effectively instigated the "law of scarcity." We all know this one: people want what they can't have and by constantly being available, you diminish your value. If every time you walked outside your front door there was a huge pile of diamonds to step over, you'd hardly see them as precious would you? The law of scarcity only makes them want you. Be around and then not around and they'll want *and* like you. I'm stating the obvious here, but liking someone is important. We talk endlessly about chemistry, passion, sexual attraction, and even more about love, yet "like" rarely gets a mention. Opposites don't attract long-term; we search for similarities in a partner. Most of us can't see the point in hanging around friends we don't like, so why do it with a lover? Liking someone is more important long-term than actually loving them. It's not just similarities in our personalities that count. If you go out with someone who looks like you, they're four times more likely to fall in love with you! "That's so true!," said a girlfriend, when I told her this trivia tidbit. "Look at my sister and her husband!"

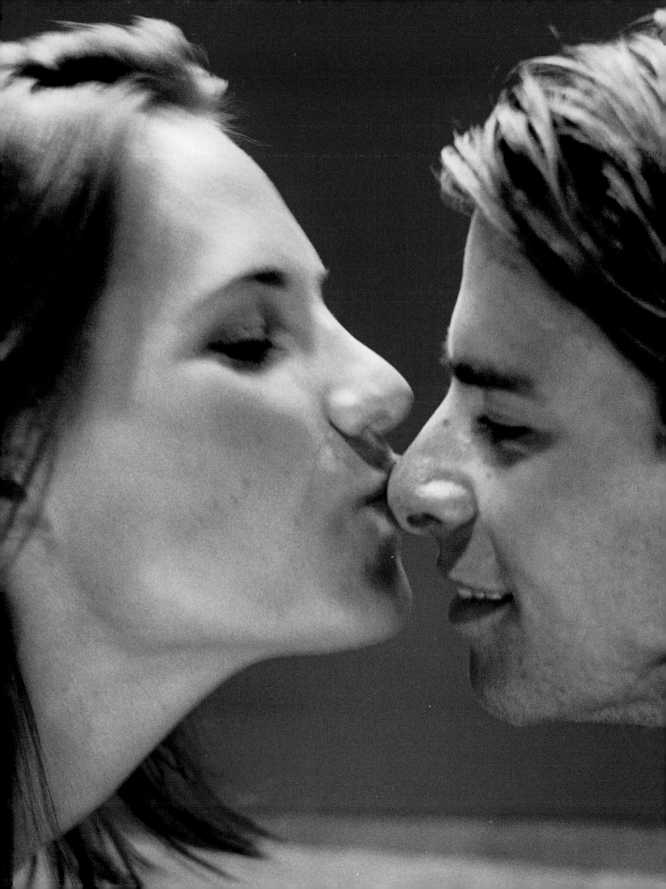

Umm—why? Lisa's sister has bleached blonde hair, freckles, and ivory skin. Her husband is Indian. "I'm not quite with you," I said carefully. "I know it's not obvious," she said, "But it's the proportion of their faces. His mother came up to me at their wedding and said 'They will be happy because they are the same. Look at them.' And it's true. They have the same features, in the same places, in the same proportions."

DON'T DO NICE THINGS FOR THEM. LET THEM DO NICE THINGS FOR YOU

If you do something nice for someone, it makes you feel good on two levels. You feel pleased with yourself and extra-warm toward the person you've just spoiled. To justify the effort or expense, we often overidealize how wonderful they are to deserve it! End result: we like the person more. When someone does something nice for us, we're pleased. But there are a whole lot of other emotions that come into play—and they're not all good. Sometimes we feel overwhelmed. There's pressure to

> PEA is secreted by **the nervous system** when we first fall in love. It makes our palms sweat, **our tummies flip over**, and our hearts race.

live up to being the wonderful person who inspired such a gift/act, not to mention pressure to return the favor. It's all even trickier if the "nice thing" comes from someone you very much like but aren't sure about yet. Got the point? When we're infatuated with someone, we're desperate to do nice things for them. You're much better off letting them spoil you.

GIVE THEM THE EYE

Harvard psychologist Zick Rubin set out to see if he could measure love scientifically and achieved it by recording the amount of time lovers spent staring at each other. He discovered that couples who are deeply in love look at each other 75 percent of the time when talking and are slower to look away when someone else dares to intrude. In normal conversation, people look at each other between 30-60 percent of the time. The significance of what's now known as Rubin's Scale is obvious: it's possible to tell how "in love" people are by measuring the amount of time they spend gazing adoringly. Some psychologists still use it during counseling to work out how much affection couples feel for each other. It's also happens to be remarkably handy information if you want to make someone fall in love with you. Here's how it works: If you look at someone you like 75 percent of the time when they're talking to you, you trick their brain. The brain knows the last time that someone looked at them that long and often, it meant they were in love. So it thinks OK, they're obviously in love with this person as well, and starts to release phenylethylamine (PEA). PEA is a chemical cousin to amphetamines and is secreted by the nervous system when we first fall in love. PEA is what makes our palms sweat, our tummies flip over, and our hearts race. The more PEA the person you want has pumping through their bloodstream, the more likely they are to fall in love with you. While you can't honestly force someone to adore you if they're not remotely interested, (They won't let you look into their eyes for that long, for a start!), it is entirely possible to kick-start the production of PEA using this technique. Try it. I think you'll be pretty impressed with the results. Give someone the sensation of feeling in love whenever they're with you, and it's not such a huge leap of logic for them to finally decide that they are!

DON'T LOOK AWAY

There was another crucial finding from Rubin's research: the couples took longer to look away when someone else joined the conversation. Again, if you do this to someone who's not in love with you (yet), you trick their brain into thinking they are and even more PEA floods into their bloodstream. Relationships expert Leil Lownes calls this technique making "toffee eyes." Simply lock eyes with the person you like and keep them there, even when they've finished talking or someone else joins the conversation. When you eventually do drag your eyes away (three or four seconds later), do it slowly and reluctantly—as though they're attached by warm toffee. This technique may not sound terribly inspired but, believe me, if done properly it can literally take your breath away. If you're too shy to gaze openly, skip the toffee and think bouncing ball. Look away and at the other person who's joined the conversation, but every time they finish a sentence, let your eyes bounce back to the person you're interested in. This is a checking gesture—you're checking their reactions to what the speaker is saying—and lets them know you're more interested in them than the other person.

PRACTICE PUPILLOMETRICS

We all know "bedroom eyes" when we see them: it's the look of lust. There's just one thing you need for bedroom eyes: big pupils. According to pupillometrics, the science of pupil study, this is the crucial element we respond to. You can't consciously control your pupils (one reason why people say the eyes don't lie). But you can create the right conditions to inspire large pupils and get the effect. First, reduce light. Our pupils expand when they're robbed of it, one reason why candlelight and dimmer switches are *de rigueur* in romantic restaurants. It's not just the softening of light that makes our faces appear more attractive, larger pupils also help. Scientists showed two sets of pictures of a woman's face to men. The photograph was identical, except for one thing: the pupils in one set had been doctored to make them larger. When shown the doctored photograph, men judged the woman as twice more attractive than when shown the real photo. It was repeated with a man's face and tested on women and gave the same result. Our pupils also enlarge when we look at something we like. Again, this can be proved using pictures. This time, researchers snuck a picture of a naked woman into a pile of otherwise bland, commonplace photographs then watched men's pupil size when they flicked through. Without exception, the men's pupils expanded on cue. This means if you're attracted to someone a lot, your pupils are probably already big, black holes. All good. To ensure this is happening or to up the effect of your bedroom eyes, focus on the part of the person you like the most. (On second thought, better make it the next best thing.)

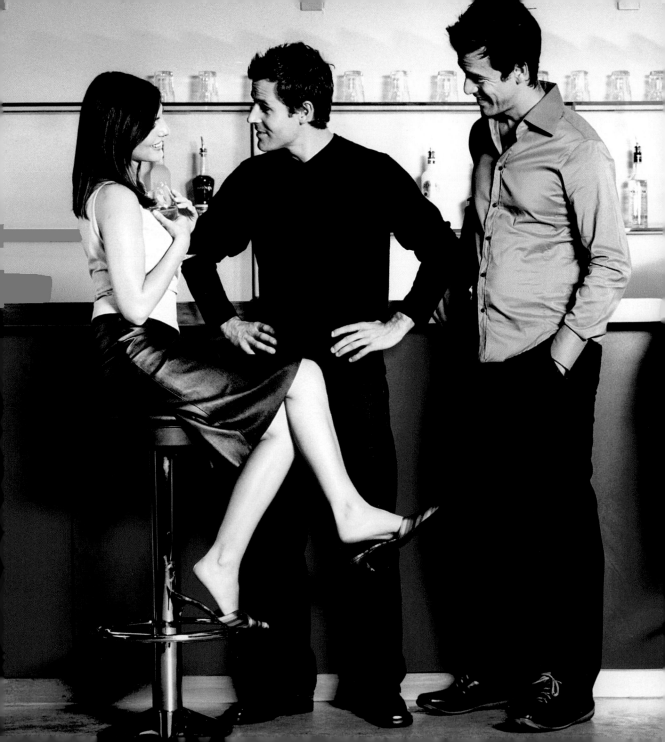

being friendly?

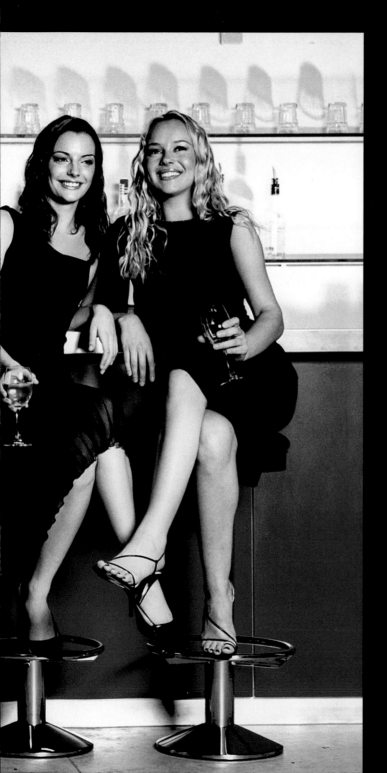

Have you been paying attention? If you have, hopefully you'll spot the clues to who's genuinely interested in whom, and on what level. Be forewarned though: initial impressions can be deceptive and all is not as it first appears when looking at this picture. Start by studying the group of three people on the left. A quick glance and it seems the girl at the end of the bar is interested in the guy in the black top standing next to her. After all, she's smiling, facing toward him, and he's leaning forward to invade her personal space. All are signs of sexual interest. Look a little closer, however, and you'll see telltale signs that the real flirting is happening between her and the tall guy in the blue shirt. His raised eyebrows give a clue. Spot an eyebrow flash and you'll know that someone's interested even before they do! Although the woman's smiling at the guy standing next to her, it's an insincere smile. A real smile fades and broadens in response to what's happening, while a fake one stays fixed. It's clear that her jaw is straining to hold this polite smile in position. She might be leaning forward, but it's toward the bar, not the guy. Other signals suggest she's not at all happy about having her space "invaded." And what about the pretty girls at the other end of the bar? What does their posture say as they look out into the crowd? Lots actually. To find out more, turn the page.

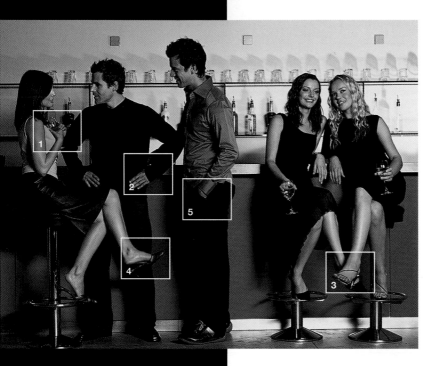

What's really

Don't ignore the obvious

- Body language is a science and a damn good indicator of someone's hidden motives, but it's not infallible. Use your common sense: do the messages you're getting from their gestures seem logical to you.

- Don't rely on one gesture only. Instead, look for "clusters"—at least three or four signals all saying the same thing.

- Trust your gut instinct. Let your body instinctively react and respond to the obvious before honing in on detail.

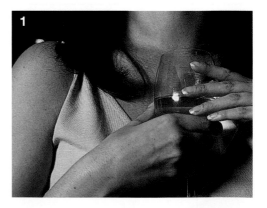

The arm barrier (1) The woman's response to the man on her right is to form an undetectable arm barrier. Holding a glass of wine or beer between you is a disguised version of folded arms. It politely but definitely says "Don't come any closer!" Unfortunately the message is blurred: her fingers wind around the glass quite seductively. It's not surprising he's confused.

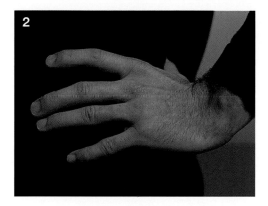

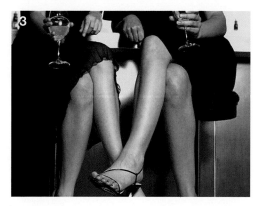

The aggressive pose (2) The hand on the hip, and the fact he's leaning forward into her intimate zone (within 6 in) both indicate this guy is aggressively stalking his prey. The jutting chin and strained neck suggest he's talking at her rather than to her. Men move into aggression flirting mode for two reasons: there's competition, or she's not responding. Both are true here.

The unspoken invitation (3) Judging by the way these two girls are sitting they'd welcome the attention of strangers. They're facing toward the crowd with relaxed, open body language. Why aren't men flocking to join them? It's their mirroring. Their bodies are almost matching images. They're obviously close friends, so to impress one, you'd have to impress both.

going on...**have they scored?**

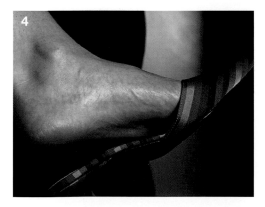

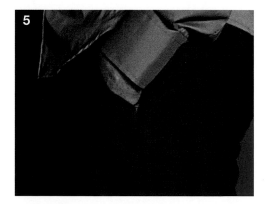

The dangle (4) Her feet give two clear clues of her true feelings. Our feet invariably point toward the person we want. While the feet of both men point toward her, it's blatantly obvious which guy she's got her eye on. Not only has she crossed her legs so both feet point directly at Mr. Blue Shirt, she's also dangling a shoe off her toes, a surefire flirting signal.

The hidden point (5) We use our hands and feet to point to the body part we most want the other person to notice. No prizes for guessing what this guy is pointing to, even if he is disguising it by having his hand in his pocket! Incidentally the other guy is also pointing to his genitals by placing his hands on his hips and pointing downward.

READ THE ROOM

Turn heads by making an entrance (see p.26), then scan the room to find who'll most welcome your attentions. Look at people's shoulders: the higher the shoulders, the tenser the person. Search for a nice, relaxed pair. Look for people standing together but staring outward: they want to be rescued so are a good bet. The groups having the best time are often the hardest to break into. Usually they're good friends who stand close together (so it's hard to muscle in), talk constantly, pause little, and laugh lots. They've little to gain by small talk with a stranger, so wait until they've caught up on the gossip and fragmented into twos or threes. Groups of strangers stand farther apart, conversation is quieter and punctuated by silences. They'd welcome you barging in. Pick your target, join them, and sparkle.

Pick up at a party...

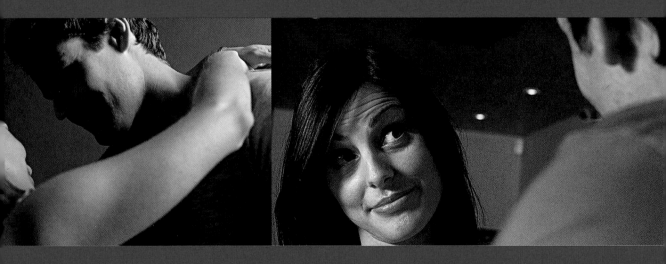

MAKE THEM WELCOME

While you're in warm-up mode, make others welcome to approach you by turning your body slightly so that you're forming an angle of 90 degrees to whomever you're chatting with. This is called standing in open formation, and it sends an unspoken, subliminal invitation for people to join you. If there are two of you, this will mean making a triangle (picture where a third person would stand, then leave a gap for your imaginary friend). When a third person does join you, you've got your triangle. If a fourth person arrives, you'll probably all form a square, before breaking off into pairs. Make sure you're in the twosome you want by immediately placing your body directly in front of the person you like and locking eye contact while everyone jostles into position. If there are five people, you'll either form a circle or break off into two triangles (and the whole process starts again.) Once you're in your tête-à-tête, stop other people from interrupting by moving into closed formation. Reduce the angle from 90 degrees to zero so that you're facing each other directly.

MAKE THEM LAUGH

Dazzle with light, frothy, fun conversation initially, then keep their interest by provoking a right-from-the-belly laugh. One minute of laughter relaxes us for up to 45 minutes! Both laughter and smiles release "happy" hormones into our bloodstream. Feel-good junkies that we are, we listen longer, talk longer, and feel warmer and friendlier toward people who inspire this feeling. If you've got a wicked sense of humor and are a good storyteller, now's the time to do it. Just be a little careful about which story you pull out of your witty repertoire. One friend once opened a conversation with a priest by talking about a bouncer who used to work at a strip joint. One of his jobs was cutting the string off tampons for the performers so they wouldn't show when they were flinging their legs around. Hysterical to most of us, not to him. Even worse though is to fall into the trap of telling jokes. I've met two people in my life who are so good at joke-telling, I laugh out loud. I suspect you're not one of them. (Sorry to be nasty about it, but seriously, don't go there unless your day job is stand-up).

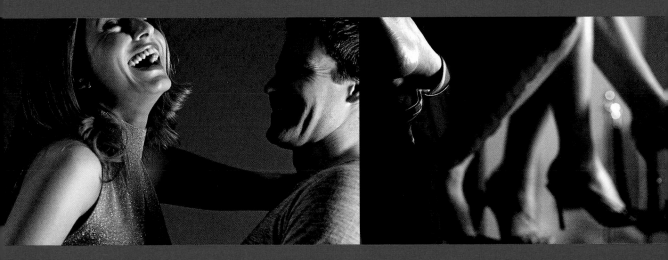

BE THE PERSON MOST LIKELY TO BE PICKED UP

- Be easy to get to. Make sure they don't have to wade through a dozen drunken friends to get to you.
- Check that your drink sends the right message. Scotch on the rocks, a pint of beer, a classy cocktail—all give clues to your personality and the kind of night you're up for!
- Look confidently around the room, meet the eyes of people you find attractive. Choose any number of eye techniques to get them interested (see pp.42–45).
- Have your hands in view. Don't hide them, sit on them, or clench your fists.
- Don't fiddle. It's OK to pree; it's not OK to shred the beer coaster.
- Cross your legs. If you're a girl: cross your legs and point them toward the person you find attractive. Hold one hand at the base of your throat. It looks sexy and it's a settling gesture if you're feeling nervous.
- If you're a man: sit like a man, with legs apart and feet planted on the floor or on the stool. Don't squeeze them primly together or cross them or you'll look prissy and girly.

IN A BAR

They're traditional pickup places, which makes bars and clubs easier in one sense— at least everyone's in the same head space. But two things work against you: alcohol and the competition (there's usually lots of it). For this reason, save the subtle come-on signals for early in the night (when people are sober enough to spot them). Later, when everyone's got their beer goggles on, judgment becomes heinously confused. When soused, some people interpret an innocent "Hello" to mean "Grope me please." Others stumble into paranoia land and need hit-on-head-with-whopping-great-steel-bar moves before they'll really believe you like them. Use the techniques on the previous page to get their attention, then once you're talking play the come-here-go-away game

Pick up anywhere…

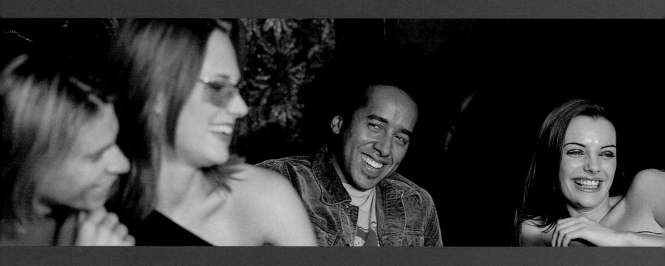

to stand out from the crowd and beat any hovering hordes. Start with clear signals that show you're interested: (come on you know how to do it by now!) lean forward, preen, smile, do lots of gooey eye stuff. Wait till they've responded by doing the same, then pull back, lock eyes, and half smile ("OK, it's clear we like each other"). Then, ever-so-casually, show slight disinterest. Look into the crowd to see what's happening, talk to other people ("Hurry up and take advantage because this offer's not going to last for long"). Just when they start to despair, turn on the flirting spotlight, and give them your full attention again. Say their name, turn so your body's squarely facing them, look at their mouth, create your own private space ("See? You'd miss me if I went away"). Just in case there's any doubt you're not the sexiest being ever to cross their path, seal the deal with a touch. Look directly at them, then run both hands through or over your hair, brushing it back from your face. ("Have a good look/Wouldn't you like to be doing this?"). Immediately afterward, touch them deliberately, while delivering a compliment. "God, you are just fascinating," as you touch their arm (safest), cup their cheek (very direct), place a hand on their thigh (call the cab).

AT A DINNER PARTY

If you're single, want a relationship, and get invited by friends you don't know terribly well to a dinner party that promises singles you don't know at all, for goodness sake go! It's the absolute BEST chance you have of meeting a long-term partner; at the very least you might find a new person to play with (and the more single friends you have, the better!). There's a trick to everyone adoring you in this situation, however (including the particular person you've got your eye on): it's called fitting in. Birds of a feather flock together and each close-knit group of people has their own way of doing things. If they speak fast and loudly, interrupt each other, hug freely, and encourage instant intimacy, you can be their new touchy-feely friend. If they speak in whispers, sit up straight, and make small talk, you do the same (then get the hell out of there). If you're desperate to impress or the group is particularly wary of newcomers, it's an idea to match verbally as well. That means agreeing with the "group" opinion and attitude. Later, when you feel you've been accepted, you can afford to be yourself and different.

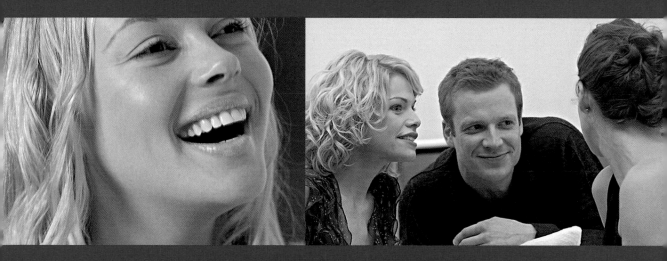

A happy, well-functioning group subconsciously protects itself by closing ranks on anyone who might alter the dynamics: interfere, criticize, or change it. There's one exception to this rule: if, upon closer inspection, your friends turn out to be just awful and the (sexy) newcomer seems to agree, bonding over a disastrous evening by running away to somewhere more private is obviously the way to go!

WHEREVER YOU ARE, BE THE BEST LOOKING ONE THERE

Now this is one of the few body language "tricks" that I find quite unseemly. It's one thing to be adept at reading other people's sexual signals and maximizing your chances of getting the best possible result from people. But this is different—it requires hanging around with people based on what they look like. (Never a terribly good idea, I've found.) If someone new meets you and you're either by yourself (nothing to contrast against) or with someone less attractive, you'll be seen as more attractive. We judge people against who they're with. What we've just been exposed to also counts. So it's probably not a great idea to be anywhere near Hugh Hefner's mansion on the night of a Playboy party.

How to pick up when you're out with friends

It's quite common these days for men and women to have a best friend who's of the opposite sex. Which is great in a "haven't we relaxed about things (and about time, too)" type of way, but not so fab when you're trying to get a date.

People look at boy/girl combinations and automatically think boyfriend/girlfriend—even when you're actually brother and sister! When I lived in Sydney, my brother and I would often go out together, completely confusing everyone. He lived two minutes up the road so we'd tend to arrive together and leave together but (as siblings do) often completely ignore each other during the middle. Once, a girl sidled up to me at a party and said, "Dump the bastard! I would!" An interesting statement at any time, but particularly if you've got no one actually to dump. "Umm, I don't quite get you," I said. "Him!," she said, pointing a finger accusingly at my brother, "Your boyfriend has been flirting outrageously with my friend!" "I know," I said grinning, "She seems really nice, actually." The girl took a step back. "Oh, I get it. You're swingers. That's disgusting!" and flounced off to inform her (rather amused) friend who already knew I was his sister, not a swinger.

You've basically got four options to stop situations like this from happening to you. 1) Ditch all friends/siblings of the opposite sex (unthinkable) 2) Wear little badges saying "I'm not with him/her." (If you're even considering this one, you're on your own from here on.) 3) Drop the "We're just friends/brother and sister" thing into conversation as soon as possible. (Recommended, but it still doesn't solve problem of how to get them talking to you in the first place.) 4) Use body language to make it abundantly clear you're both related/friends and available. (Guess which I'm going to recommend.)

There's an obvious place to start in your quest to keep your friends and score yourself a lover: have a chat to them. Let's be honest here: it's quite handy having opposite sex friends who are single, and we're all a bit guilty of trying to keep them that way. The best kind of friends will openly admit this, maybe even own up to feeling possessive and deliberately flirting with you if someone else threatens to muscle in. And sometimes it feels great on your end, too! The "I don't want you but I don't want anyone else to have you either" game can be flattering. Not quite so cutesy when it blows your chances with someone you really like.

If your friends are notorious for ruining your pickup chances, let them know that although you adore their friendship and would NEVER let a partner come between you (their real fear), the fact is you do want a relationship and them flirting with you and/or being possessive is sabotaging

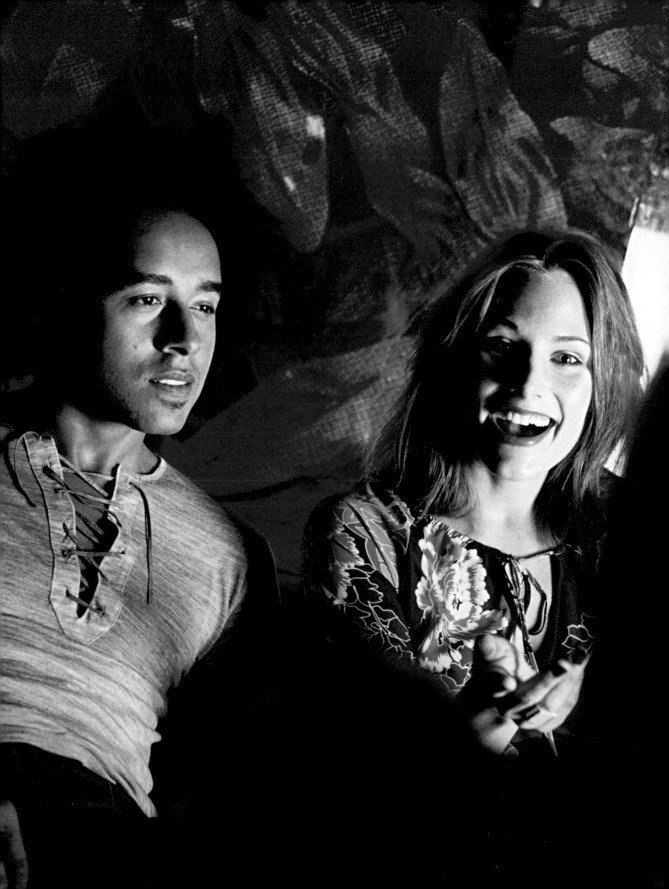

things. Having said that, none of these body language adjustments is going to make your friends feel enormously special. So if it's just you and a close friend out on the town, I'd strongly advise you tell them what you're up to. Here's your "keep it friendly, but not flirty, when out with friends" checklist. Do a mental run-through each time you nip to the bathroom to make sure you're getting it right.

THE CHECKLIST

- **Put some space between you** Don't lean in close or sit close together. Don't touch too much and restrict touches to nonintimate zones.
- **Laughing lots is fine but make sure it's loud laughter rather than low and intimate** Avoid long periods of intense eye contact, and keep glancing out into the crowd.
- **Keep your body turned slightly away from your friend and facing the crowd** If this feels too rude, turn your upper body toward them but keep your legs and feet pointed toward the crowd. Others will receive the subliminal message that you're not trying to create an intimate zone, so it's safe for them to intrude. It's called standing or sitting in open formation (see p.136).
- **Have breaks in conversation** When you do, let your gaze travel around the room. This says "I'm open to meeting new people."
- **Don't glue yourself to their side** Get away from your friend or the group as much as possible. Chat to other people. Go to the bathroom lots, taking your time going there and back. Offer to go to the bar and get the drinks—friends are much more likely to take turns than couples.
- **Use your eyes to invite people to join you** One universally understood "chat up" sequence is to look, then look away, then back again. Do this twice. Turn your body to face them.
- **Get friends to put in a good word for you** If your friend is the confident, friendly type, this is how they can help immeasurably. When they next go for drinks, get them to take a detour past the admired one and say something like "My friend thinks you're gorgeous!" or "How embarrassing! My friend won't take their eyes off you!" along with a big smile. This reassures the potential date on two levels: the words "my friend" mean that's all you are and the smile says you haven't got a hidden agenda. You're not likely to be encouraging matchmaking if you've got them earmarked for yourself!
- **Add a broad smile and hold eye contact for four seconds next time your eyes meet** If the eye contact is returned and it's smiles all around then it's time to step things up. You've got two choices here: approach them, or encourage them to approach you. Whatever you do though, make it fast because they'll be doing some fast thinking too at this point…
- **Make the move yourself** It takes exceptional courage, or complete and utter arrogance and/or stupidity to hit on someone blatantly when it's just two people and they're both of the opposite sex. Even if you've sent clear signals that you're not with your partner, they still can't be entirely sure. You might be single and out with a friend—or you might be some sleazeball who gets off on eyeing up other people in front of your partner. Or they've got it wrong, and you're not giving them a look at all. See how it can all go horribly wrong? I'd especially opt for making the move yourself if you're male. Plenty of women still think it's the "man's job" to make the first physical move by closing that crucial distance. A liberated, confident woman won't think twice about crossing

the floor but others might think it'll look desperate or "unladylike" if they come to you.

- **Use your friends as an excuse** Hanging out with friends does have advantages—you never need to worry about opening lines. All you need to say is something like this: "My friend Jane/ John is sick of listening to me go on about how pretty you are/what a great smile you have. They've made me come over and say hello even though I'm sure you've probably got a billion boy/girlfriends already." The beauty of this intro is all in the implications: it delivers a compliment but it's indirect so less embarrassing. It makes them feel the friend is on their side. By saying you were "made" to come over and you're there to say "hello" means you're unlikely to hang around if you're not welcome. Finally, by suggesting they're already taken gives them a nice easy way out if they're not interested. All they need to say to get rid of you is "Thank you, that's a real compliment! Trouble is, you're right. I actually do have a boy/girlfriend." They're off the hook, your ego's intact, everyone's happy. Well, as happy as you can be when you've just been let down.

Let's be honest here: **it's quite handy** having **opposite sex friends** who are single, and we're all a bit guilty of trying to **keep them that way.**

- **Bringing them back to your friend** It's working and you're chatting away happily? If you've gone to them and you're out with just one other person, stay chatting for 10 minutes or so before bringing them back to meet your friend (agree beforehand that you'll both have to survive as best you can for this period). When you do rejoin, include your friend but pay special attention to the new person. Again, you'll be seen as a rude so-and-so if you don't alert your friend to what's going on first, so consider working out some sort of code. Maybe two tugs on the left earlobe means all's going well and they should think about giving you privacy. If after half an hour they return to find you're still chatting away intimately (or have become decidedly more intimate), they should bow out gracefully. I know if seems harsh, but as long as you don't abuse the privilege, it's reciprocal and neither of you do it constantly, most people are more understanding than you think. There'll be plenty of chances to involve them later—this is about giving you the best chance to make a good first impression.

- **If you've gone to them and you're out with a group...** wait about half an hour before rejoining. Then, give them the choice, say "I might just go over and explain to my friends where I am. Do you want to come with me and meet them or would you prefer to wait here?" If they're brave and volunteer to be introduced, do it with a flourish so they feel important, let small talk take over for a few minutes, then block so it's just the two of you again, using your body to create a little private space around you. Lean in close. Put your arm up. Monopolize them. Don't get drawn into side conversations that don't include them. Keep your body turned toward them. Maintain strong eye contact. In other words, make it abundantly clear that they're your prime focus.

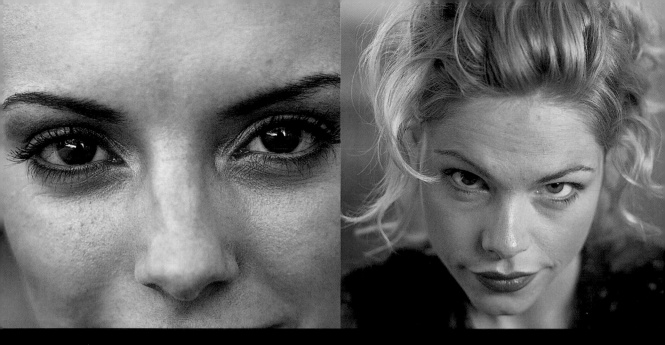

Eyes **right**

It's virtually impossible to connect and communicate with someone without eye contact—let alone flirt or fall in love. The real reason why superstars wear sunglasses at night isn't to look cool, it's to hide their emotions. Clearly revealed here is excitement (shiny eyes, top left), hostility (top right), honesty (bottom left), and stress or total boredom (an eye shutout, bottom right). A lifted eyebrow (main picture) is a facial question mark: oh really?

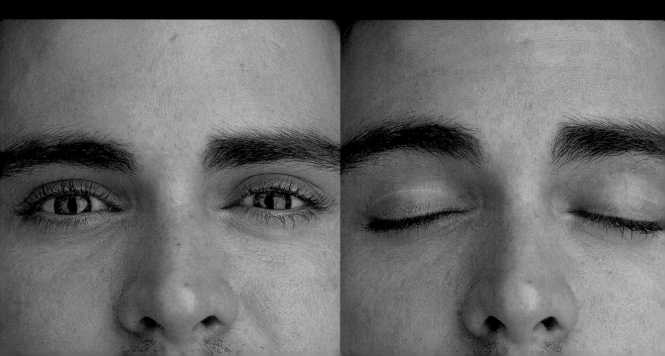

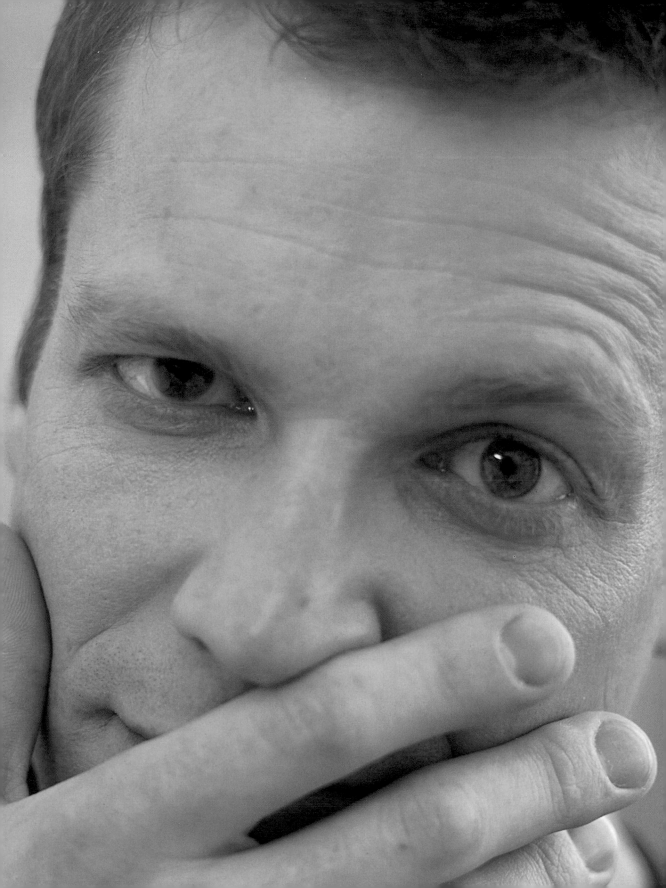

FLIRTING FIX-ITS

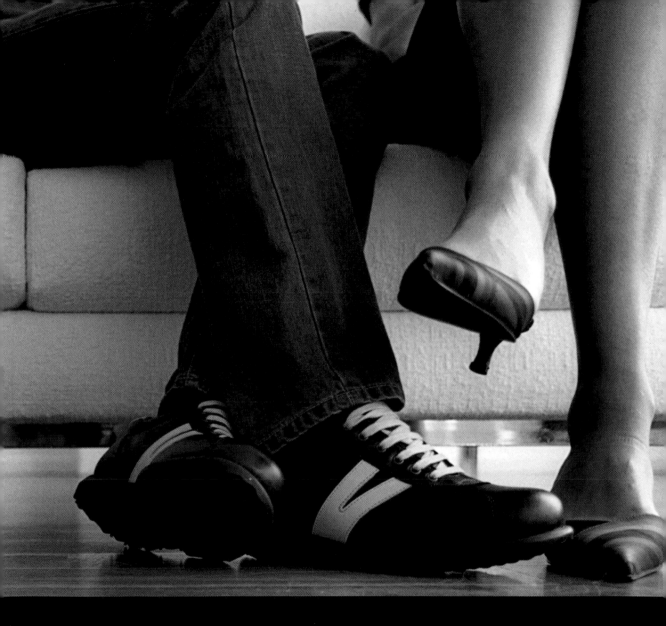

How to spot a bad bet, **when to back off** so you don't make
a complete fool of yourself, and general troubleshooting,
volume adjustment, and **unraveling of mixed messages**

Crossed lines
I thought they were interested but now I'm not so sure…

One minute it's going swimmingly well, the next not so great—even worse, you can't quite pinpoint why. The change is subtle, but you're getting the distinct impression they're losing interest Are you being paranoid—or astute?

If someone loses interest, they start de-courting: flirting in reverse. Instead of using their body to show interest, they'll start using it to show they're not interested, usually, by doing the opposite to what they were doing before. Imagine all the flirting techniques we've talked about filmed, then played backward. That's de-courting. Instead of staring into your eyes, they'll break the gaze and turn their eyes away from your face. Instead of leaning forward, they'll straighten up or lean back. Instead of facing you squarely and standing close, their torso twists away and they step backward to create distance.

Shame you weren't at a dinner party I went to once, because you could have seen the de-courting dance illustrated in technicolor. Maxine, a friend of mine, threw the party for two reasons: 1) For me to meet Mike, her fab, new boyfriend 2) For me to meet his equally as delicious single best friend. "Meet Mike and Steve," she beamed on my arrival, pushing two gorgeous blond men in my direction. Yum Yum! Forget dinner. Shooting her a conspiratorial wink of approval as she disappeared into the kitchen, I sidled up to Steve and launched a full-frontal flirt attack: a veritable whirl of eyelash batting, hair flicking, meaningful looks, touching, charming, and general flirting. I couldn't have looked more adoring if he was the captain of the Starship Enterprise, about to save the Earth. When Maxine finally reappeared and we sat down to dinner, I practically tackled another guest to sit next to him. Mike ended up on my other side and, figuring I'd better make an effort to get to know the boyfriend, I made polite chit-chat, all the while glancing back over my shoulder to dart provocative "I'll be back" looks to Steve. What a fantastic guy! I tried to catch Maxine's eye again to give another "Wow!" look, but strangely she glared at me. Like really, really glared. Wow! "Maxine doesn't seem very happy," I whispered to Mike. "Are you two having a row?" "No," he said, looking a bit confused. "Well, I don't think I've upset her. I don't know her very well though…" Protectiveness of Maxine flared. What did he mean he didn't know her very well? And shouldn't he be more concerned? "God, I hope I haven't done anything wrong," he continued, "Because Mike would kill me. He's besotted with her." "What do you mean Mike? You're Mike," I said, dread building in the pit of my stomach. "No, I'm Steve," he said, "Did you mix us up?" Oh dear God. You want to see flirting in reverse, you should have seen me that night. I backtracked so fast, I left skid marks. Maxine thought it was hysterical, but Mike (the real one) was just plain confused. Even now, he eyes me with suspicion, not sure how I'm going to behave. One minute dripping all over him, the next acting like he's Quasimodo with a hygiene

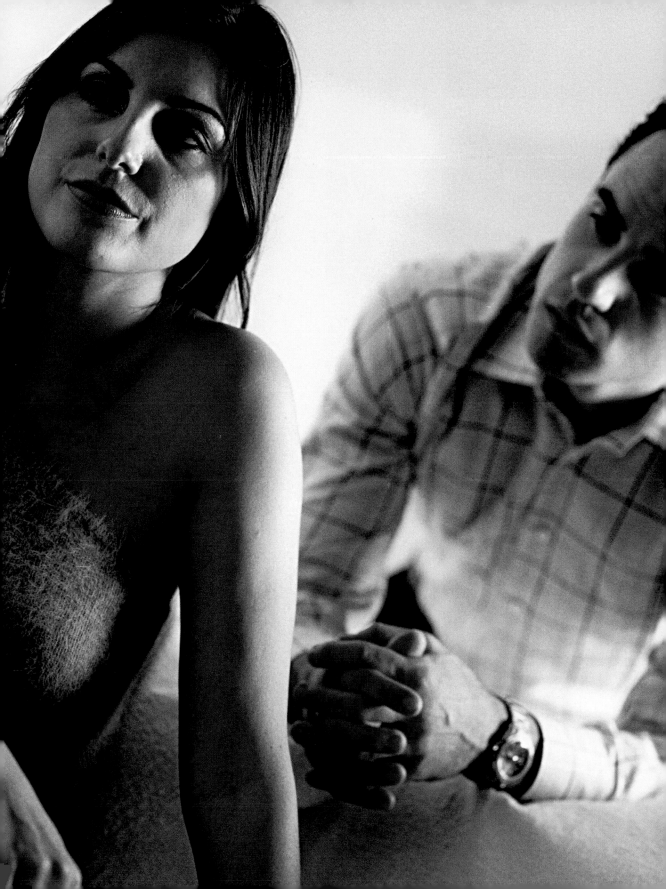

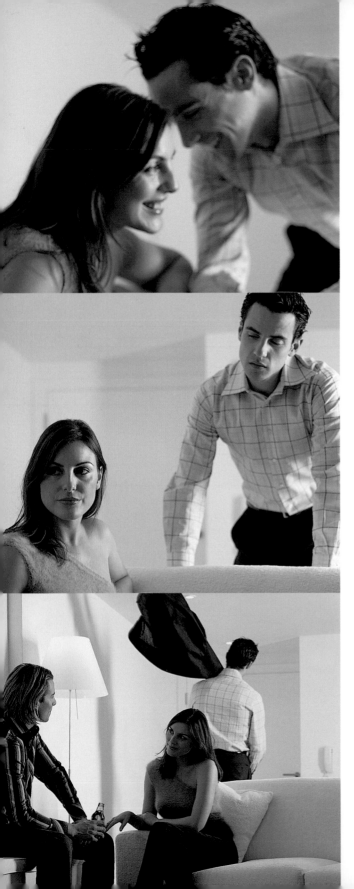

problem. That's de-courting, and if someone's doing it to you, it definitely means they've lost interest. Now let's look at what you may have done to cause it…and whether it's fixable!

WHAT COULD HAVE GONE WRONG

- **You didn't apply the Rule of Four** Don't assume someone's interested in you unless they show a minimum of four separate, positive signals simultaneously and these signals are directed at you. You're looking for what's called "clusters"—lots of body language gestures saying the same thing. The friend who greets you with a huge smile, outstretched arms, sparkling, excited eyes, and dilated pupils is pleased to see you. That's a happiness cluster—four signals that usually mean someone is happy occur together and are aimed at you. The mistake some people make is interpreting body language signals solo. They spot an eyebrow flash and think "Aha! They want me." One hour later a foot points toward them and they take that as another sign of interest. Ten minutes on, the person starts preening, and they start mentally debating which champagne cocktail to serve at the wedding. Taken separately and aimed generally, body language gestures mean little. Always apply the Rule of Four.

- **They've changed their minds** You know what it's like: the person looks delicious from the other side of the room, then you start chatting and their breath knocks you out/they mention their passion for plane-spotting/the fact that Mommy still approves all their dates. How we appear isn't always how we are, and some people back off fast if you're not what they thought you'd be. It happens to everyone occasionally and there's not much you can do about it. If it happens often, however, ask a good friend: how's my voice and content? (Is your voice off-putting, do you swear too much, are you coming on too strong, too quickly?) Does my appearance and image fit my personality?

- **They're playing mind games** This is the really annoying part—even if you read their body language right and they were practically climbing into your lap, people play games. Sometimes, we flirt with everyone else in the room except the person we really want. Sometimes it's because we're too shy to march right up to them and hope by flinging our hair around in close proximity they'll notice us. Other times it's to make them jealous. If you're the pawn they're pushing around the come-here-and-chase-me chessboard, it can be very confusing (not to mention humiliating once you discover what they're up to!).

- **Something has triggered a reaction** All it takes is the wrong song to come blasting through the speakers and the person who was happily flirting away can suddenly go cold. Why? It reminds them of an ex who shredded their heart and their self-confidence. Things like this are largely out of your control. After all, how are you supposed to know his ex gambled away their life savings, so your funny story about losing in Vegas takes on ominous undertones? If someone suddenly makes an abrupt mood change and you're pretty sure you've done nothing to cause it, chances are this is what's happened. If it's really obvious and you've got nothing to lose, it's worth asking gently, "Are you OK? You seem a little faraway. Have I said something to upset you?" They might confess and even if they don't, you've shown you care and that alone can be enough to shake them out of it. If, on the other hand, they shake their head and clam up even more, forget it (and probably them for the moment). Probing further won't get you anywhere.

More than just friends?

How do you let a friend know you've got the hots for them? Try these three tests.

- Next time you say goodbye, hold their hand and pull them close, then give their hand a squeeze as you're kissing them. Plant a kiss, dead center, on the lips, making it last 2–3 seconds. Pull back slightly, keeping your face close to theirs, then kiss them again very quickly (but hard). Pull back, look them straight in the eye, squeeze their hand, and let go. If they're interested, it'll give them the green light. If they're not, it'll seem like an overly affectionate goodbye. It's OK if they look a bit stunned; they're digesting the message you've sent. Check out their pupil size (the bigger, the better). Do they look flushed and red and put a hand to their mouth or bite their lips? (All good.) If they quickly meet your eyes, they're checking they've read the situation. You've created "a moment" when anything seems possible.

- You tried it and still no clues? Ask a good friend to make discreet inquiries ("Do you know my Mom always said you and Jenny would make a great couple. Weird isn't it, thinking of friends as lovers, but have you ever thought of going out with her?") Often, this type of love remains unrequited simply because it's never stated.

- You've given it one or two tries and still nothing? Know when to give up. I had a friend who turned me into a quivering heap just looking at him. Quite unlike me, I (sort of) let him into my heart though I knew he'd hurt me. Alistair openly admitted he was a commitment phobe, but constantly flirted with me and the idea of a relationship. He played emotional yo-yo for about three months. He's still a friend and still tries to play the game, the difference now is I don't even notice. Know when to put someone firmly in the "friend" basket and leave them there.

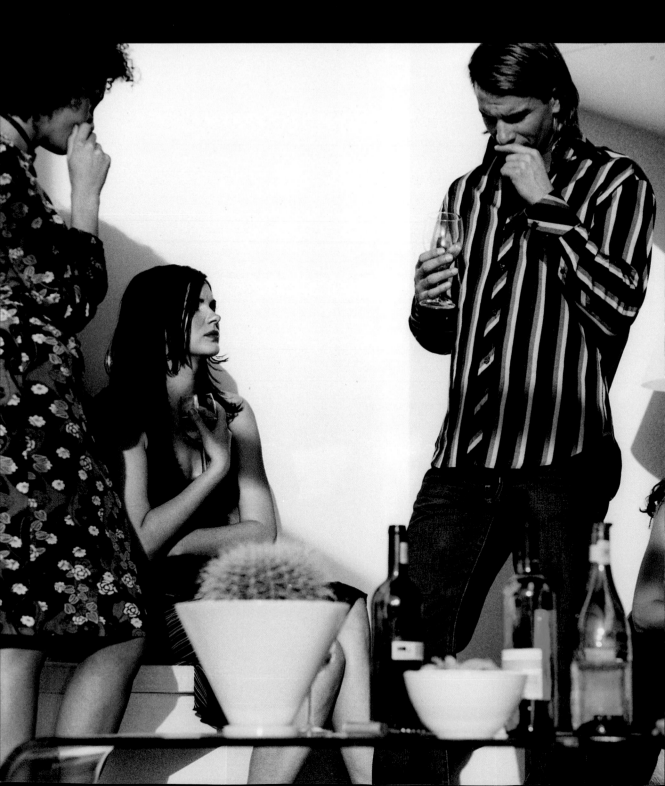

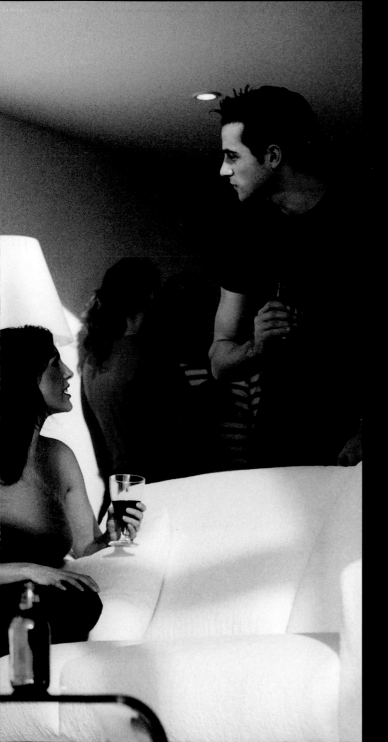

Want to get away with a lie? Stop feeling guilty about it. Our body language rarely gives us away if our mind's convinced the lie's not going to hurt anyone. White lies are easy; big, bad ones aren't. When forced to lie, we get scared. Fear makes us sweat, our breathing becomes uneven, we talk less, swallow more, speak slower, and fiddle with things. Our throats become dry, feet flex inside our shoes, and our voices raise in pitch. Lying is stressful and hard to get away with because it involves faking emotion and expressions. Most people know avoiding eye contact is a giveaway, so a good liar will look you straight in the eye. Trouble is, they overdo it, to the point where their eyeballs dry out, causing them to blink furiously and…Gotcha! Another problem with playing pretend: it's hard to get the timing right. Watch the person who's genuinely surprised by the party thrown for them and it comes and goes quickly. A faker will hold the look of surprise much longer. Feigned emotion appears slower than normal (we mentally compose the expression first) and disappears abruptly (it's a strain to hold it). Other signs are more subtle. See the group of three on the left? The girl standing up just had a one-night stand with her (seated) best friend's boyfriend, the man in the striped shirt. Meanwhile, the man standing behind the couch is struggling to hide his own secrets from his suspicious girlfriend. What gives them all away? Turn the page…

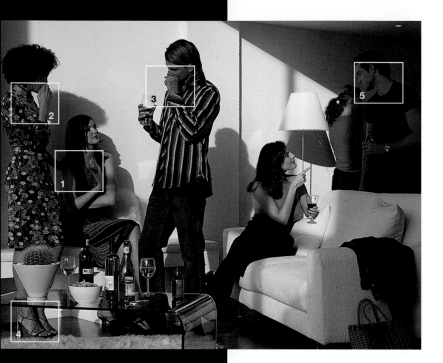

A liar:

- **Never forgets. Most of us, when asked to recall something, get a few details wrong. A liar has a story already made up. Asked to repeat the story over and over, it'll stay word perfect.**

- **Visibly relaxes once they think they've gotten away with it. Change the topic and they'll seem instantly happier and often laugh nervously.**

- **Can't control micro-expressions. FBI agents are taught to look for them as they accuse someone, because real, raw emotion flashes across our face before we can compose our features.**

A scenario of

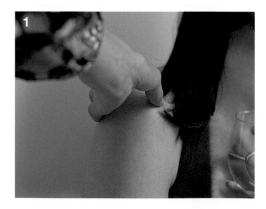

The defensive barrier (1) Her guilty friend comforts her from a distance, but this girl subconsciously realizes things aren't quite right—her body's moved into a defensive position. She's crossed one arm over her stomach and the other upward, protecting her heart. The slightly slumped body posture and blank expression also suggest unhappiness.

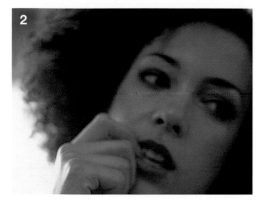

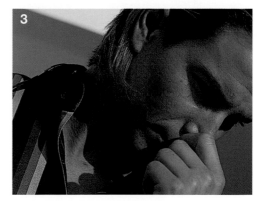

The guilt giveaway (2) We often touch our mouths when anxious or guilty and this girl is literally zipping her lips, trying to stop any giveaway words from slipping out. This combined with the troubled brow, downcast eyes (to avoid meeting anyone else's), and the left knee pushed slightly forward are all signs she's hiding something.

The Pinocchio pose (3) It's not a fairy tale: your nose really does grow when you're telling a lie! Our body reacts to stress by pumping extra blood through the body, causing our noses to swell and grow by a fraction of a millimeter. You can't see it with the naked eye, but it makes the nose feel slightly tingly and many people respond to the sensation by touching it.

deceit . . . the crucial clues

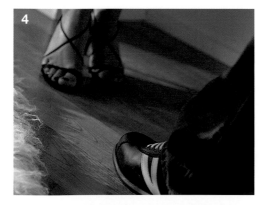

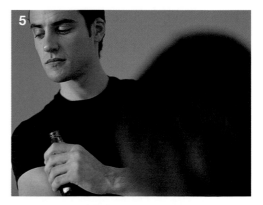

Suspicious mirroring (4) The fact that their feet are pointed toward each other shows that the naughty twosome's bodies are still attracted, but their brains have comprehended the fallout if they're found out. They also mirror each other with their bodies: they have the same knee pushed forward, and are both holding hands to their faces and looking down.

Eyes right (5) Most of us look to the right when we're mentally constructing something (making something up) and to the left when we're trying to recall information. It's a quick, instinctive movement that is almost impossible to fake. Judging by this, and the fact that he's using the couch as a shield, this guy is not being altogether honest with his girlfriend.

Spot a **sexual triangle**

When I first moved to London and was saying goodbye to my much-adored brother at Sydney airport, it suddenly hit me that I was going to live on the other side of the world, and I burst into loud, body-racking, hiccupy, sobs. "Oh God," I sobbed. "I'm going to miss you so much. I don't think I'll ever get used to it." "Trace, you'll be over it the minute you set eyes on that duty free shop," he said kindly. "I'm not that shallow!" I said huffily. Ten minutes later, there I was, trying to choose between the silvery Chanel eyeshadow (very glam!) or the cute little Dior palette with the most divine pinky-pearl (more practical). Tears miraculously dried. Most of us do survive when parted from loved ones. Brothers,

> Are they **standing the same**? Do they sip their drinks at the same time? If so, they're **bonding on a subliminal level.**

though missed, are contactable by phone. Hearts, though broken, nearly always heal. But there's one betrayal that delivers a near fatal blow, and that's when your partner runs off with a close or best friend. Losing your partner and the person whose shoulder you'd have sobbed on, is a particularly poisonous double dose of betrayal. Research shows people who heal quickly and without too much scarring have one thing in common: they suspected something was going on, even if they didn't voice their fears or both parties denied it. Knowing we'd recognize the signs if it happened again gives us the faith to take another risk. Which is why this piece is about how to tell if you're in the middle of a sexual love triangle, by looking closely at body language and behavior. Here are the basics:

- **It could be about to happen** If your boyfriend sits between you and the friend you suspect, he'll sit close to you, but his body and gaze will turn toward her. She'll angle her body toward him, usually with legs crossed in his direction, and lean forward with her upper body. She may rest her hand at the base of her throat, fingers splayed. Often, subconsciously, you'll pick up an unwelcome vibe and lean in closer to him and your friend, to involve yourself in the conversation and establish your connection to both. If you haven't done it consciously, do it now. Smile lots at your friend, make direct eye contact, and throw a quick but genuine compliment her way. Then make a subtle ownership gesture to your boyfriend, like kiss him on the cheek while simultaneously squeezing his hand or leg. This reaffirms your relationship to both of them, pushing the guilt button so hard, it can't help but hit home how underhanded what they're contemplating is.
- **It could have been going on for a while** Watch for all the typical courting gestures because all will be evident, if done in secret. She'll briefly touch his leg under the table while you're not looking, shoot loaded looks and make meaningful eye contact whenever you look away. To catch

them at it, turn your head so they can't see your eyes (and appear to be looking in another direction) but you can still see them. Pretend to be absorbed in a task and watch for signs. Betrayal is often fueled by lust (anything forbidden becomes appealing) so you'll see lots of autoerotic touching (both of them will start caressing their own lips, necks, arms whenever together) and preening (smoothing or adjusting clothing or hair to make sure they look their best). Watch for brief but sexy, wry, intimate smiles and pay particular attention if the conversation turns to sex or relationships. The guilty will react one of two ways: clam up and look intensely uncomfortable, or play flirty little games with each other (and you). If she's single, she might say "Sex? What's that! It feels like I haven't had sex for a million years but God, I'd just love to do it right now." This will be followed up by a quick look at him from under her lashes. If she's attached, she may be over-attentive to her partner and overflirt with him instead. A favorite is to kiss her boyfriend, while maintaining eye contact over her shoulder with a potential or secret lover so he can see what she's like in action/recall what it's like to kiss her. She's effectively saying I wish you were him.

- **They're attracted to your partner but aren't doing anything about it** Take notice if friends who used to adore your partner, suddenly aren't as friendly. If your best friend Hugh is now weirdly quiet around your girlfriend Emma, it's often because he knows something you don't (your girlfriend's playing around maybe) or he's after her himself. If we want someone we shouldn't, we tend to become less chummy. We're scared we'll give too much away if we're palsy, so we create distance. Along with the new aloofness can come slightly aggressive teasing. He's resentful he can't have her, so he'll subconsciously seek to decrease her "value" to him by belittling her. Sometimes people are so successful at doing this they not only cease to find the forbidden person attractive, but they also start to wonder why their friend still does, dropping "You could do better" hints.

- **Your partner's not interested** They seem slightly embarrassed whenever the person is around, fixing you with desperate, devoted looks. They're trying to transmit a message with their eyes: "I want you to realize he/she's hitting on me and I don't like it but don't want to hurt you by telling you because this person is your friend." They'll also close themselves off from the person: turn their body away from them and toward you, refuse to make eye contact, and avoid being near them in situations where there's close body contact (like sitting next to her in a crowded car).

- **It's bad news if they start mirroring the person's behavior** Are they standing the same? Talking at the same volume level? Do they sip their drinks at the same time? If so, they're bonding on a subliminal level. Which way are their feet and hands pointing? Even if his torso faces towards you, a foot pointed squarely and firmly one pace in her direction may mean he's attracted. Test you're right: move closer to your partner, mirror their movements, smile warmly at them, drop your voice to a low, intimate level to talk about something that clearly links you, and push an imaginary hair out of their eyes. All are ownership gestures that say "Back off!" but it's your partner's reaction that is important. If they go stiff and move or lean backward when you snuggle in, refuse to be involved in an intimate discussion, and turn their body away from you when talking to the "suspect," the writing's on the wall. Watch their eyes, too. Sometimes, they'll lean in with their head to listen while you're whispering in their ear but keep looking at the other person. It's the equivalent to the kissing scenario: I wish it were you, not my partner, whispering in my ear!

Getting completely sloshed nearly always tops the list for Oh-my-God-I-can't-believe-I-did-that disaster dates. But there are plenty of other ways to unwittingly put someone off. Check that you're not guilty of these common dating mistakes.

1. RESTING YOUR CHIN IN YOUR PALM, ONE ELBOW ON THE TABLE

Not good: The message you're sending when doing this: I'm so bored/tired, I haven't got the energy to hold my head up. It's also a pose we assume when objectively summing someone up since it discourages any physical contact. (You try touching or hugging a friend with one hand stuck under their chin—it feels weird!) Assume this pose after a friend's just told you devastating news and they're likely to be horribly offended (and rightly so). If you're not completely confident of your looks, you'll also have a tendency to sit like this. People who like their faces move them around, letting people admire them from all angles (lots of women hold their hair back off their face, to let men have a good look). By looking out from behind your hand, you're hiding most of your face from view. Not a good move. Not even if you're a supermodel.

Try this instead: The only way you can possibly get away with cupping your chin in your palm, is to be truly besotted. Couples in the lovey-dovey honeymoon stage will often simultaneously adopt this posture, slumped on the table, gazing into each other's eyes. In this situation, the posture switches from showing boredom to adoration. In every other case (excluding 12-year-olds gazing at a popstar poster and those at the beginning of a sexy, sultry love affair) it's to be avoided at all costs. There is no substitute pose—just get those hands away from any type of supportive position.

2. AWKWARD HANDS

Not good: Wringing your hands, sitting on your hands, balling your hands into tight fists, clutching onto a drink/bag/menu so tightly your fingers go white, fiddling, shredding labels/napkins—all these signs signal nerves and anxiety. Putting your fingers in your mouth (but not in a good way) or biting your nails says, "I'm insecure and need reassurance." Later on, I'll suggest sexily sliding a finger suggestively into your mouth as an autoerotic gesture. But there's a huge difference between this and practically shoving your whole hand in there—which is what we tend to do when we're under pressure. Psychologists say it's an unconscious attempt to revert back to the security of breast-feeding: sucking our fingers is the equivalent of sucking on our mother's breast. A bit Freudian, I know—but this one actually does make sense. As kids, we replace Mom's breast by sucking on our thumb, and adults often break that habit by biting their nails. (Interesting how most of us bite our thumbnail more than any other.) Theory aside, it looks unattractive. Stop it. Now.

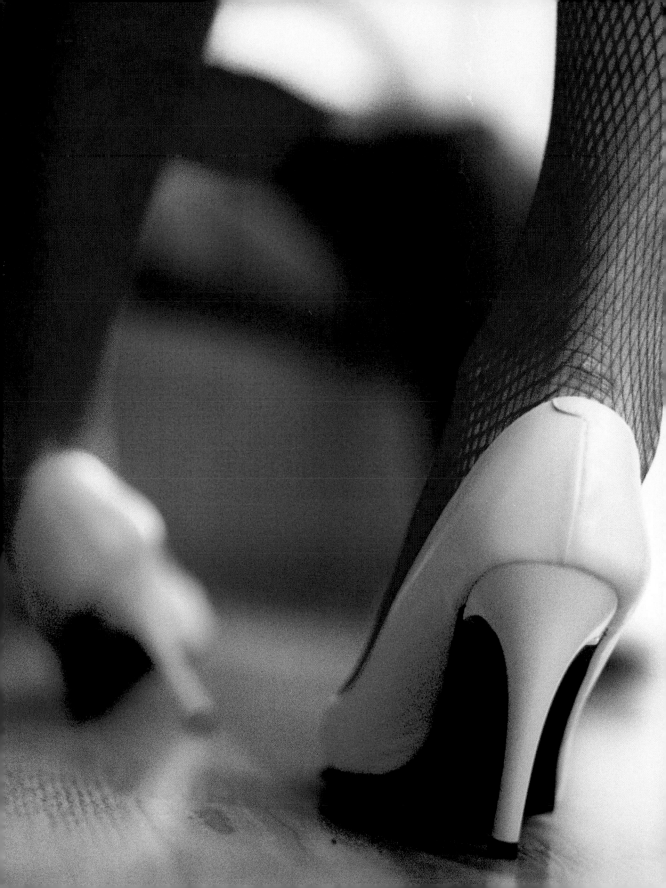

Try this instead: "But what do I do with my hands?" is one of the questions I'm asked most often. Shy or nervous people don't move around much, so whatever position they adopt with their hands can look forced. Any position will look awkward if you hold it for too long. The trick is to practice two or three different hand positions in front of a mirror and switch between them. Start by sitting down in front of a table (how you'd usually sit when out to dinner or in a bar). The first thing to remember is to keep your hands in view—in other words, stop sitting on them or shoving them between your knees. You do it because you don't want people to see they're shaking, but people also sit on their hands when they're lying and hiding something, so it also looks decidedly shifty. Get them up and on the table! Rest your forearms on the table, keep your arms open (but not ridiculously

Flirting **faux pas...**

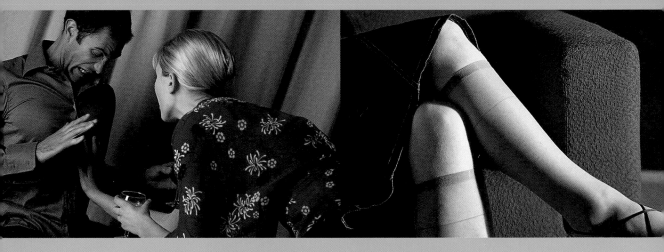

wide) and just let them drop forward. They've probably dropped so they're about 18 inches apart, your palms are facing toward each other, fingers relaxed but slightly curling inward. (If your arms are dangling in space, drop them closer to the table. Actually resting on the table is fine, too.) Now, pretend you're talking to someone (yes, good idea to do these exercises when everyone else is out) and move your hands around, gesturing to back up what you're saying. The positions you want to continue using are those where your hands and arms are open and relaxed, the front (palms) rather than the back of your hands are facing the person you want to impress. It's better to avoid crossing your arms, though it's usually OK if they're relaxed and loose, if you're leaning forward with your elbows resting on the table (just make sure you don't stay in this position or clutch your arms tightly). A really good trick if you're feeling nervous on a first date dinner is to "steeple." Rest your wrists on the table palms facing each other, then spread your hands out, splay your fingers slightly, and press your fingertips together. Touching fingertips has a calming effect and it also makes you appear more confident. We steeple our hands when we're certain of what we're saying or about to say and have no doubt it will be believed: we're in control of the situation. We tend to steeple with fingers pointing upward while we're talking and fingers pointing downward while we're listening. Women tend to favor low, unobtrusive steeples, usually pointing down; men tend to steeple higher with fingertips pointing up. In general, the higher the steeple, the more confident you are.

Once you're done with seated hand gestures, stand up in front of the mirror and see how they all translate. Keeping your hands relaxed, palms toward people, steepling—all work while standing as well. The trick now is to move them around a lot. Use your hands to illustrate your words—wave them about if you feel passionately about something, lean forward to touch the person you're talking to, preen a little (smooth your clothes, brush your hair back). Do anything other than stand in the classic I'm-terrified position of clutching onto your drink with white knuckles, holding it in front of you as protection.

If **you're the type** of person who stands so still at a party people start **hanging their coats on you**, making any sort of movement's got to be **a major improvement.**

3. NOT MOVING
Not good: Standing or sitting so still, you look like a rabbit caught in the headlights of an oncoming car.
Try this instead: "People on the move" is a phrase used to describe interesting, dynamic people. Take it as a literal translation. Lots of shy, nervous, insecure people stand very still. Lots of enthusiastic, outgoing, passionate people move around a lot. Note the emphasis on "lots" because this by no means applies to everyone. If you're the type of person who stands so still at a party people that start hanging their coats on you, making any sort of movement's got to be a major improvement. By all means practice and perfect all the "good" body language gestures and postures listed in this book, although they won't get you anywhere if you simply adopt one position and freeze in it all night. Instead of settling on one way to hold your hands/sit/stand, why not master three or four variations? That way you can switch between them all, looking far more relaxed and confident and much less contrived.

Help! It doesn't seem to be working!
Are they interested or aren't they?

Some people send out such clear sexual signals, it couldn't be more obvious if they had "You're gorgeous. Want a date?" printed on their t-shirt. Others fall truly, madly, deeply in love with a good friend and remain so their entire lives without giving a single clue of their affections.

The majority of us fall somewhere in between: sometimes we're great at flirting, other times not so great. Unfortunately, most of us tend to be outstanding flirts and body language decipherers with people we don't particularly care for and lose the plot entirely when faced with someone we do! There are a million tips (well, lots anyway) scattered throughout this book that are designed to help you show you're interested without laying yourself on the line. But what if you've done all that and are still none the wiser? What do you do if you think someone's interested but you're not completely sure? Is there a way to test if they're flirting with you? There certainly is! Read on…

HOW TO TEST IF SOMEONE IS FLIRTING WITH YOU

- **Check your own body language** Are you sending clear signals you're interested in them? Could be you're sending out mixed signals and they're mirroring you? Be honest with yourself: What are your motives for getting together with this person. What are your true feelings? Is your body leaking what your brain is telling you (you sort of like them but aren't quite sure?)
- **Send at least five distinct signals to show you like them** The best: 1) Stand close and face them directly. 2) Make lots of eye contact 3) Keep your body language generally open (uncross everything and relax your shoulders) 4) Smile and keep the conversation light and sexy 5) Touch them (in a safe place, such as their arm or shoulder).
- **Apply the Rule of Four** Check that they're sending four positive sexual signals simultaneously and that they're all directed at you (see p.150).
- **Think about the circumstances and context** Where are you? If you're at a work function, they might be scared to show they're interested for fear of being seen as unprofessional. What's their mood? If they seem nervous and distracted, it could be because it's their party and they're worried about their guests. If they've just landed the job of their dreams, they'll be euphoric and much more flirtatious than usual. If they've just lost it, they're hardly in the mood for frivolity. What's their relationship history? The person who's just been dumped will react one of two ways: 1) By clinging to the nearest replacement like a drowning man 2) By punishing all women/men and behaving like an idiot. How much have they drunk? If they weren't so enthused but are now acting as though you've mysteriously transformed into the latest pinup, it's

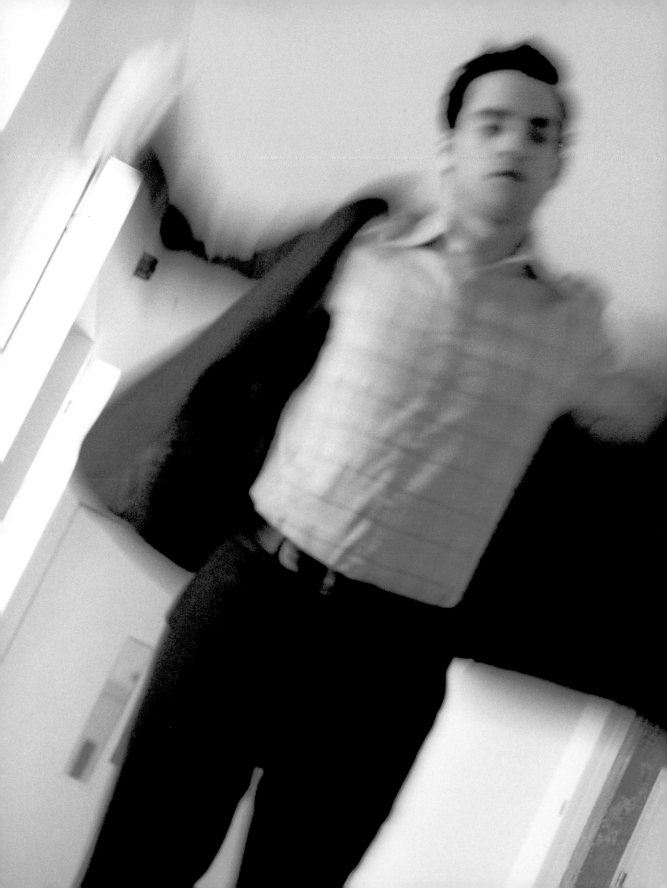

probably the booze talking. Beer goggles make everyone look good. Combine this with The Closing Effect—people rate others more attractive as the night draws to a close—and I wouldn't read too much into their declarations of devotion. If you want a fling or one-night-stand, go for it. If it's a relationship you're after, hand over your phone number, but don't wait around for the call.

- **Think logically** Say someone's leaning in, smiling and attentive to you but also pretty obviously scanning the room. It could mean they're mildly interested but keeping their eye out for someone better—or it could mean they're waiting for their partner but enjoying a sneaky flirt with you in the meantime. Ask: "You seem to be looking for someone. Are you waiting for anyone or trying to find your friends?" If they are attached, chances are they'll own up; if they're just being rude, you've drawn attention to it. They'll either decide you're worthy of their full attention, or make their excuses and disappear in the direction of the nearest blonde. What if someone's giving you great eye contact, their feet are pointing toward you and their whole

> The guy who finally **gets to chat** to **the girl of his dreams** will want to flee and stay simultaneously.

body's pivoted in your direction but they've got their arms tightly crossed? Crossed arms might mean they're defensive, nervous, or anxious—or it might mean nothing at all (they always stand that way or they're a bit cold). Whichever, it's in your interest to get those arms uncrossed. Studies show simply having our arms crossed can evoke negative emotions, because it creates a physical barrier. Try handing them something—like a drink or something for them to hold, so they're forced to uncross their arms, and see if it makes a difference. If it doesn't make them more open to you, it's probably just a habit to stand like that. Dismiss the negative signal and believe the positive.

- **Listen to what they're saying** If what they're saying seems to contradict what their body language says, believe the body language. Mouths lie, body language rarely does—but you do need to apply some common sense. If someone's flirting like crazy but smoothly evading all your attempts to find out if they're taken, assume they are. Their body isn't lying because they do want you, but that doesn't mean they're free to follow up on it. If their body language is contradictory, it could be because they've got the urge to do two things at once. The guy who finally gets to chat to the girl of his dreams will want to flee and stay simultaneously. He's terrified he'll blow his chances so wants to run away, but is desperate to win her over so stays put. Because he can't do both at once, he'll do one, then the other, which transforms into swaying, shifting from foot to foot, pointing his feet in the direction of the exit, jiggling his legs, putting his hands on the side of his chair like he's about to get up, but maintaining adoring eye

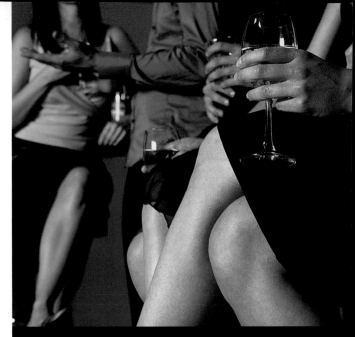

contact, etc. If you're getting mixed messages, this is what's usually happening. Ditto the girl who describes herself as happily married, while unconsciously slipping her wedding ring on and off her finger: there's definitely trouble in paradise. The best bet is someone whose words and body language convey the same message: they've got no hidden agendas.

- **Test they're flirting with you, by flirting with them** If you've worked through the checklist and are pretty sure they like you, up the stakes by very obviously making a play. Whisper something in their ear and let your lips touch their cheek as you're doing it, pull back and make gooey eyes. Use every trick in this book to make it obvious you think they're sex on legs. If they're interested, they'll mirror you by increasing the intensity of their flirting. If they're not—or they're flirting without intent (having fun but aren't planning on taking it further)—they'll tone down their advances or stop flirting completely. You made it clear it was crunch-time—make a move or move on—and they've responded.

- **If you're too shy to superflirt, pull back a little instead** Stay friendly but be a little less flirtatious. Start them wondering if they've misread and maybe you're not interested after all. If they are, they'll turn up the volume and start making obvious advances to reel you back in again and keep things flirty. Try doing it this way: once you've connected with someone, back away slightly to create a little distance between the two of you, but maintain eye contact. This issues a clear invitation to enter your intimate space zone and poses a silent question: Are you interested and are you going to do anything about it? If they step forward into your space on their own accord, the answer is a definite "Yes!".

How to spot who's available

- **Available body language** doesn't mean the person is available to you legally or morally, it just means they'd like to be. Your body doesn't care if you're still in your wedding dress on the way to the honeymoon suite. If it spies someone it wants to have sex with, it'll still send out the signals!

- **Singles** regularly scan the room for potential partners, notice newcomers, and tend to keep their faces half-turned toward the crowd. They're in attraction mode: body language turned outward. The attached and happy focus their posture inward, toward their own group. They're less likely to look up when people enter the room and if they do, they glance up briefly.

- **Shy people** often appear unavailable because the same body language which makes them blend into the crowd, also equals disinterest (avoiding eye contact, slumped shoulders, bodies turned away). Introverted people don't send out available signals because they're convinced you wouldn't respond anyway. If you're interested, lavish loads of compliments and see if they start to spark up.

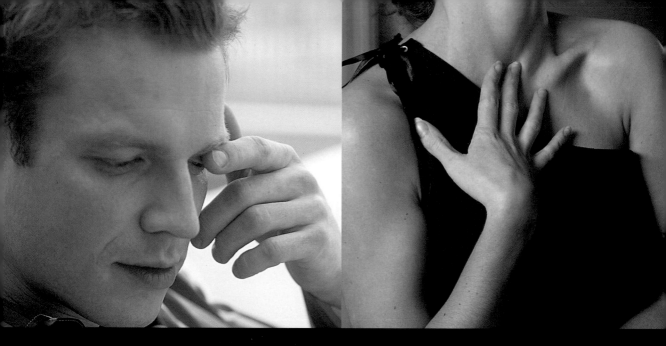

Point the way

We point to what we want, or what we want others to pay attention to. Here we see examples of wanting to sleep (finger trying to close eyelid, top left), feigned innocence ("You can't possibly mean little ol' me?" top right), sexual attraction (feet pointing toward female, bottom left), and a classic "notice me" gesture (one hand points to highlight the other, which is clearly pointing toward whoever is opposite, bottom right). The man in the main picture, opposite, points not only with his finger but also by winking, and with the tilt of his head and mouth.

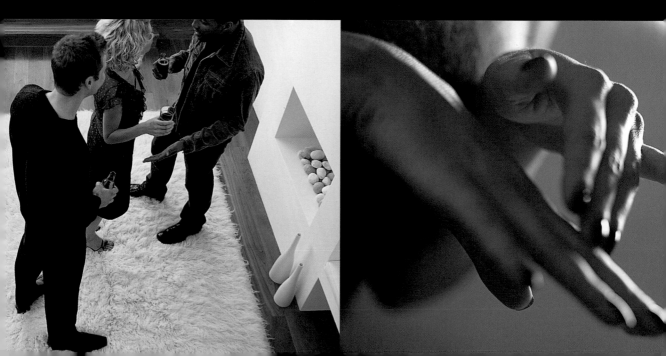

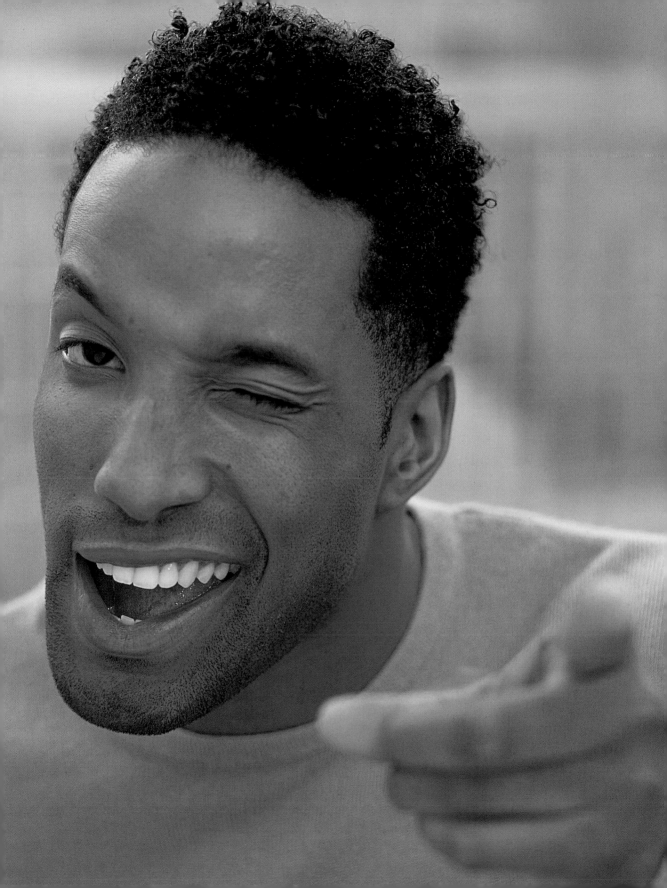

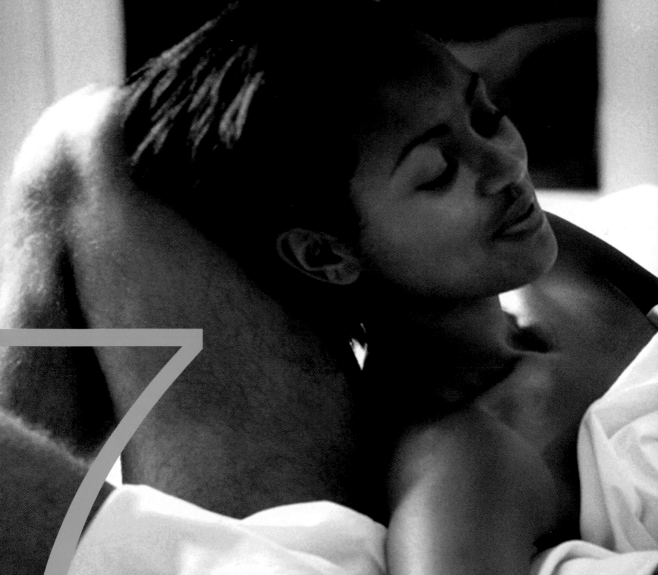

7

SEDUCTION STRATEGIES

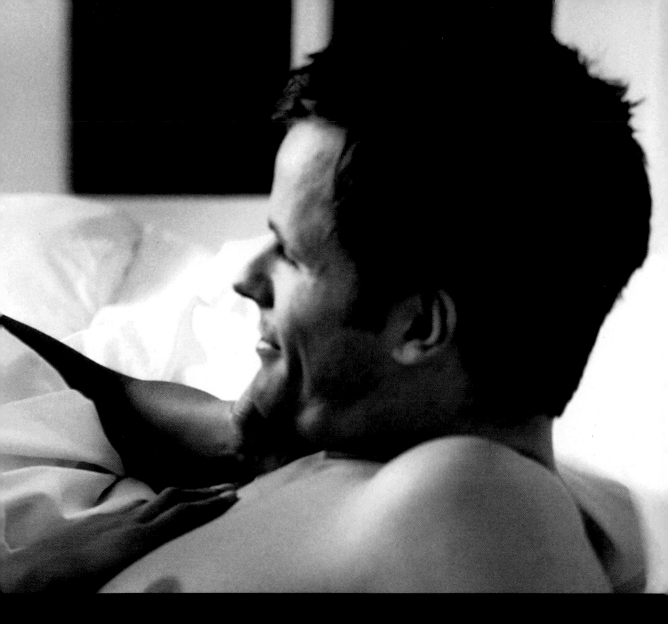

The secret signs they're ready for sex and tips on how to deliver exactly what they want. Plus, how to make sense of the **morning after madness** and figure them out from **their sleeping style**

You've done your homework and all that flirting stuff's paid off. Now, here you are face to face with a real-life version of your naughtiest fantasy. Gulp. What to do now? Keep reading, that's what…

US sexpert Barbara Keesling believes that anticipation is the key to creating explosive sex. She's all for teasing and tormenting until your partner can't even look at you without turning pink with passion. I have to say, I agree with her. Barbara coined the phrase "touch and tease" for a series of calculated seduction ploys designed to knock a potential target to their knees in a nanosecond (and I don't mean to propose). I've taken Barbara's idea, given it a twist, thrown in lots of autoerotic touching (touching yourself where others would love to), and come up with some X-rated versions of the original. Some "touch and (now) torments" work better on men, others on women. I've divided them accordingly but feel free to pick 'n' choose if you think your target's an exception!

THE WARM-UP (YOU'VE JUST MET)
This works whether you're sexily squashed on a sofa or standing in a bar in the middle of a crowd. It also works no matter what stage your relationship is at. The only proviso is you need breasts— hence why this one's for her, not him!

- While he's talking, cross one arm loosely across your waist and support the elbow of the other arm by cupping it in your hand. Now lift the supported arm until your fingers touch your chest. Splay your fingers and lift your hand so just the tips of your fingers touch and simply stroke your collarbone lightly, back and forth with your fingertips for a minute or so. Maintain eye contact the entire time and let your hand rest there when you're finished. Too vampy? Here's the **Cheat's version:** Instead of stroking, simply hold your hand there.
- The next time you laugh, throw your head back to expose your neck and as you do so move your hand to the hollow of your throat. Really, really slowly, let your fingers slide down your throat toward your breasts. Stop just where your cleavage starts (or should, depending on how well endowed you are!) and let your fingers rest there, dangerously close to the breasts themselves. Keep your fingers there as long as he is talking, but when you begin talking, remove your hand (it makes it seem less contrived and attention-seeking). He'll be fascinated because your hand is where he want his to be, and you're giving him an extra incentive to keep on flirting.
  Cheat's version: Rest your fingers at the hollow of your throat instead of your cleavage.

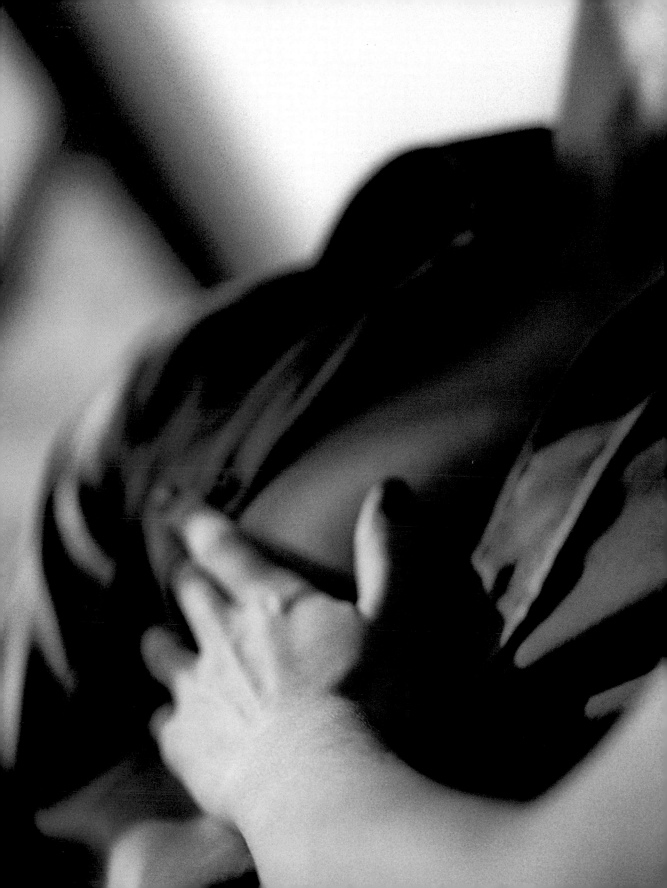

- Imagine what it would be like to kiss this guy. Make a little movie in your head, then drop your head, but lift your eyes to look at him. Now slowly stroke your bottom lip with your index finger. Thoughts of kissing him puts a wicked glint in your eye; distractedly touching your mouth hints you are indeed thinking about something racy; the lowered head adds little-girl-lost vulnerability. A lethal threesome! After a few minutes, say something like, "Sorry, what were you saying? I got a bit lost there." It's crucial with this one that you maintain eye contact or he really will think you drifted off through boredom.
  Cheat's version: If you can't bring yourself to stroke your bottom lip, look at his mouth instead.

HOT STUFF (YOU'RE DOING THE BUSINESS)

Plenty of couples are great at playing tease games in the beginning but stop the minute they start having sex. They figure once you've both had your wicked way, the pretense of the chase is over.

The **hottest session** you've had so far was **in an elevator?** Try whispering this in their ear just as their parents greet you **for lunch.**

Wrong! Sustain sexual tension by capitalizing on what's been, what's happening now—and what more there is to come. If anticipation is the name of the game (and believe me, it is), all the following will help you score:

- **The past** If you're not both practically passing out at the memory of your last sex session at the beginning of your relationship, then something's wrong (you need to lay your hands on a great sex book rather than each other). For most people, those early sessions are distinctly memorable because you're trying everything together for the first time. Think of one word that describes each session (the location, the position, or the particular body part you focused on) and you have a "trigger" to use for instant erection/arousal. The hottest session you've had so far was in an elevator? Try whispering "elevator" in their ear, just as their parents greet you for Sunday lunch. Or "tie me up—again" as you board a packed train. Triggers will propel them straight into fantasy land—choose places where you can't act on it and you've set up a sexual recall system that will make your last encounters seem even hotter than they were in reality.
- **The present** Don't just kiss her goodbye in the morning with a peck on the cheek. Hint at what's to come later that night by cupping her face in your hands and indulging in a full, five-minute make-out. Or hug her from behind while she's brushing her teeth and watch your hands caress her breasts in the mirror. Better still, grab her arms and put them around you as you're brushing your teeth then, with your hands over hers, use her hands to fondle your

body. She watches from behind as you run her hand over your chest, tummy, then follow the line of pubic hair downward ("Look what you've done to me") to masturbate for two exquisite minutes (bet she can't help continuing even when you've stopped directing her hand!) An even sexier goodbye/hello for later: as she's about to leave, lift her skirt, pull her panties to one side, and give her oral sex for 45 seconds. Just when she's thinking "Forget work, I'll be late," you stop abruptly, giving her nothing more than a sly smile.

- **The future** Here's a secret (not): men tend to escape into fantasy land if real life sex isn't hot enough for them. It's no reflection on you, by the way, just a bit of a boy thing. So instead of getting all huffy about it, next time surprise him by not just listening to his fantasies but also helping him to develop them into full movie-length plots. Make it clear that you're curious about what turns him on, though aren't (necessarily) going to want to translate anything into reality. But the one thing you can promise is you won't judge. Get him to confess to his favorite fantasy, then ask questions. Lots of them. He's gone for the classic girl-on-girl scenario? Ask "What am I wearing?/What's the other girl wearing/What does she look like?/What's her name?/Is she a lesbian or are we both bi-curious?/Are you watching?/Is she making love to me or me to her?/Am I looking at you?/Am I secretly wishing I was with you or lost in the sensation of another woman's tongue?/What's happening now?/Who's touching whom?/Am I embarrassed?/What would happen if I now asked you to join us?" I suspect you don't need to be a body language expert to see the effect your words are having…

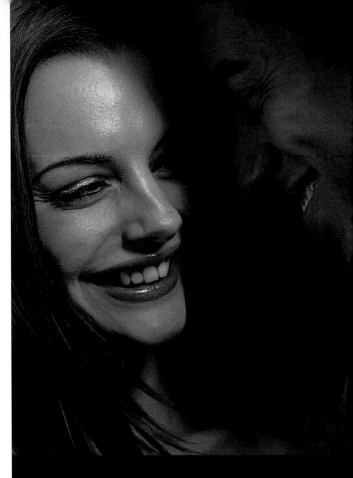

The rules of tease
- **Don't rush anything** If you do it correctly they're not going anywhere.
- **Don't be hard to get**—but don't be too easy either. A good tease doesn't promise what he/she won't deliver; it's the question of when that adds the tease factor.
- **Don't cheat** Your face reflects every thought in your head. Think sexy and you'll look it— even if you're discussing what color to paint the bathroom. Think about what color to paint the bathroom and the huskiest blow-by-blow description of future pleasures completely loses its impact.
- **Relax your mouth** Mouths give away tension. Keep lips slightly parted and imagine you're about to be kissed.

This entire book is designed to lead you to this moment. You've learned how to package yourself, make an entrance, attract attention, spot who's interested, and respond accordingly...well, now it's Crunch Time. Time to put your money where the pout is. How do you make the transition from all-out flirt mode to serious seduction? Simple! Read the signs that he's ready for more, then watch his body language to ensure you give him exactly what he wants.

SECRET SIGNS HE'S READY FOR SEX...
- He's touching his face more than usual.
- He's holding his head high.

Make every **man want you...**

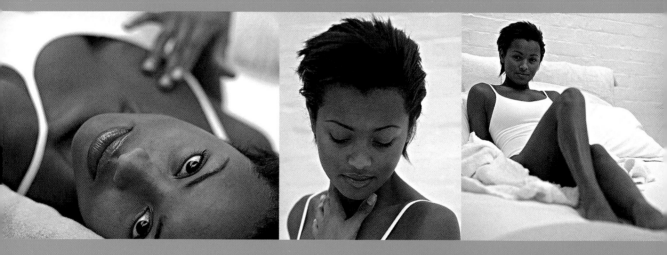

- His eyes appear shiny and moist.
- His pupils are large and dilated.
- His sentences are short and half-finished and he's breathing quickly.
- His thighs tense and his hips start moving in a subtle thrusting motion, suggestive and deliberate.
- His lips are red and swollen.
- His nostrils flare.

GIVE HIM EXACTLY WHAT HE WANTS
Well, well—you're finally doing it! Here are some hints to guarantee a smooth ride (ahem).
- How do you tell if you're really satisfying him? Whatever you do, don't rely on the hardness of his penis! If he's nervous (and who wouldn't be when they finally get to bed a sex goddess like you!), he's focusing way too much on his erection. As a male friend put it so perfectly, erections are like riding a bike: stop and think about it too much and the whole thing goes wobbly. Instead,

watch and listen for other, more reliable, signals that he's intensely aroused. Is his breathing quick and shallow? Is his skin flushed and pink? Are his lips parted?

- Pay attention to the distance between your bodies. If he's moving closer and pressing hard, he wants it deeper/harder/a more deliberate touch. If he's pulling away from you, you're being too rough or fast (or he's just about to lose control and doesn't want to give in just yet).

- Some guys love women to play innocent in bed; others want their favorite porn film reenacted. Do both of you a favor by not reading too much into his particular penchant—it's mostly out of his control. Our sexual psyches are programmed from a very young age. He's innocently playing in the back garden as the next door neighbor sets up a nice little stocking fetish simply by hanging up the washing and inadvertently offering him a glimpse of hers. He won't remember his first sexual stirrings becoming all mixed up with staring up Mrs. Darrington's skirt, but he will get an absurd amount of pleasure from watching you prance around in a garter belt.

Turn undressing into an art form. Look like you're in your own little world; meanwhile, **stay completely body aware** so you look gorgeous!

IF YOU REALLY WANT TO MAKE HIS DAY...

- **Be body beautiful** Turn undressing into an art form. Look like you're in your own little world. Meanwhile, stay completely body aware so you look gorgeous!

- **Be selfish** Treat him as a tool simply for your pleasure. Straddle him, pull your panties to one side and use one hand to direct the head of his penis so it rubs against your clitoris. Have a gloriously self-centered orgasm, then lower yourself onto him during the last stages—not to put him out of his misery but to make your orgasm last longer. (Believe me, he won't complain.)

- **Be bossy** You call the shots and start and stop the action by changing the pace and the place. Jump on top, then off again, then lead him into another room and another position.

- **Be brazen** Most women aren't comfortable being exposed—dare to be different! Show him you're proud of what you've got. Instead of being shy and closing your legs when he's admiring the view, spread them as wide as you can. The truly secure maintain eye contact as they're doing so...

How do you know if a woman wants sex? It'd be a lot easier if your girlfriend were a baboon! Unlike her shy human equivalent, the female baboon blatantly advertises when she's horny. During ovulation—when she's most likely to get pregnant and feel turned on (also true for humans)—the area around her genitals turns bright red. Just in case her mate doesn't get the message, she crouches in front of him, waving her butt in the air. While I doubt your girlfriend will wiggle her butt so blatantly, let's be honest, she is wiggling it. And there are other signs too, albeit a little more subtle.

SECRET SIGNS SHE'S READY FOR SEX
- Her eyes seem glittery and sparkly.
- Her cheeks change color—she'll blush and glow, then go pale again. Her pulse is racing.

Make every **woman melt...**

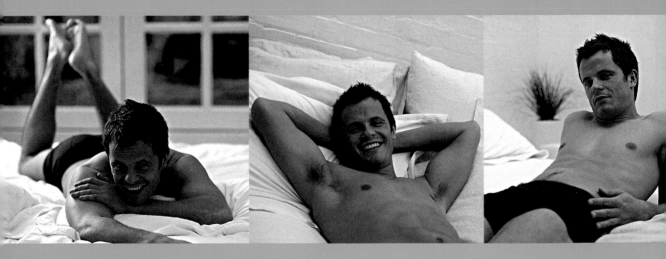

- The muscles of her whole face appear tight and toned. Her cheekbones seem more pronounced than usual, and there's a flush of color or slight rash on her neck, shoulders, chest.
- She's stroking her neck lots.
- She keeps looking at your mouth.
- She's touching her mouth and lips with her fingertips.
- She's smoothing her skirt down over her hips to accentuate the curves/tucking her thumbs in the waistband of her pants/jeans and pushing them down to show off her tummy/hiking her skirt high to show off her thighs.

GIVE HER EXACTLY WHAT SHE WANTS
- Admit it: you love hugging the remote control for the TV. Well, now you're going to do the same with sex. Just as you switch channels to control what's on the screen, you can switch body parts to control the level of her desire. Switching sexual channels not only reduces any chance

of desensitization (if touch is constantly concentrated in one area, the skin stops sending pleasure signals to the brain), it adds an element of surprise and teasing, and keeps her hovering in that almost-but-not-quite-there preclimax zone. Switch between four basic channels: the visual channel (pull back and drink in her body with your eyes, hold eye contact during sexy bits—the couple who watch each other, stay together); the mouth-motivated channel (talking dirty, kissing, biting, licking everywhere); the flesh-on-flesh channel (skin-on-skin, touching-at-every-possible-point; the touch channel (hard, soft, barely grazing her flesh with your fingertips, whole-hand massage, grabbing, squeezing, inserting your fingers, rubbing, kneading).

- Swap between all four channels to build excitement to a peak, but watch carefully to see which she seems to like the most. Then settle in to fine-tune your technique. The next session, start and finish by concentrating on her favorite channel, but continue to throw in plenty of variety and varied technique until it gets to the point where she simply can't choose among them...

Admit it: you love **hugging the remote control** for the TV. Well, now you're going to **do the same with sex.**

IF YOU REALLY WANT TO MAKE HER DAY...

- **Make her beg for it** Push her hand away and say "You can't touch me until I tell you to." Take off all of her clothes and leave all of yours on. Alternatively, take off all of your clothes and let her fellate you, but this time tell her she's not allowed to remove even her jewelry. If you're giving her oral, take regular breaks and detour back up to tongue her belly button, licking your way back down again. Then stop completely and ask, "How badly do you want me to finish?"

- **Make her cry** —out loud. A lot of women are dreadfully quiet in the bedroom, terrified that even the odd moan will somehow seem "slutty." (I mean, what would you think? That we're enjoying ourselves? How dreadful!) Give her permission to be vocal by encouraging her to let you know how she's feeling ("If you feel embarrassed telling me in words, just groan when you like it and keep quiet when you don't."). Women are natural people pleasers—you'll be the one blushing in front of the neighbors.

How scent and taste affect our libidos

We spend a lifetime planning outfits for that first date—even longer dissecting and analyzing every word spoken and gesture made afterward. While it makes perfect sense to package yourself as attractively as possible, once your bodies get intimate, it's in the lap of the gods. How we smell and taste to each other can determine whether you become an item—or walk away wondering what the hell went wrong.

THE SMELL OF SEX

Few people say "It was their smelled that hooked me." but very often it's the truth. Scents are decoded in the brain by the olfactory bulb, the part also responsible for memory, which is one reason why smell can attract us to people we'd normally cross the street to avoid. If your first sexual thought centered around a teacher who wore a musky perfume or aftershave, that particular smell and sexual attraction become linked. Years later, this might explain why the man with Elvis hair, bow-legs, and bad beard does it for you: he's simply wearing a musk-based fragrance. The olfactory center instantly reacts to the pheromones of every person you like. Pheromones are the scent version of a fingerprint: each of us has a unique, natural, undetectable smell. A blend of intoxicating ingredients —including chemicals released when we're aroused—our pheromones are also influenced by things like how oily our skin is and how much we perspire, along with mundane factors like what we've eaten, drunk, and how much exercise we've done. The end result of this olfactory melting pot is released from apocrine glands, located in our "warm" spots: armpits, groin, mouth, nipples, back of knees, wrists, and palms.

What happens when you meet someone you find attractive

The brain receives "Wow!" signals and on cue, pheromones release. Then the olfactory centers of each of you get together and have a chat to see whether it's worth it to take things further. Now here's the part that really makes you want to slap on the deodorant (don't—it masks the natural process): if the smell isn't right, there'll almost certainly be no desire. The olfactory center doesn't care if this is your first date in years or the best proposition ever, if the smell isn't right, it'll never feel right. Doesn't matter how good this person looks, if the OC's say it's not a happening thing, forget it!

MAKE IT WORK FOR YOU...

- **Wear layers of clothes** so you can peel off the minute you feel hot. Wear cotton clothes that "breathe" and wash them often. Our skin can't breathe under tight, hot clothing, which means phermones get trapped, and instead of working for us, start to do the opposite (i.e., phew!).

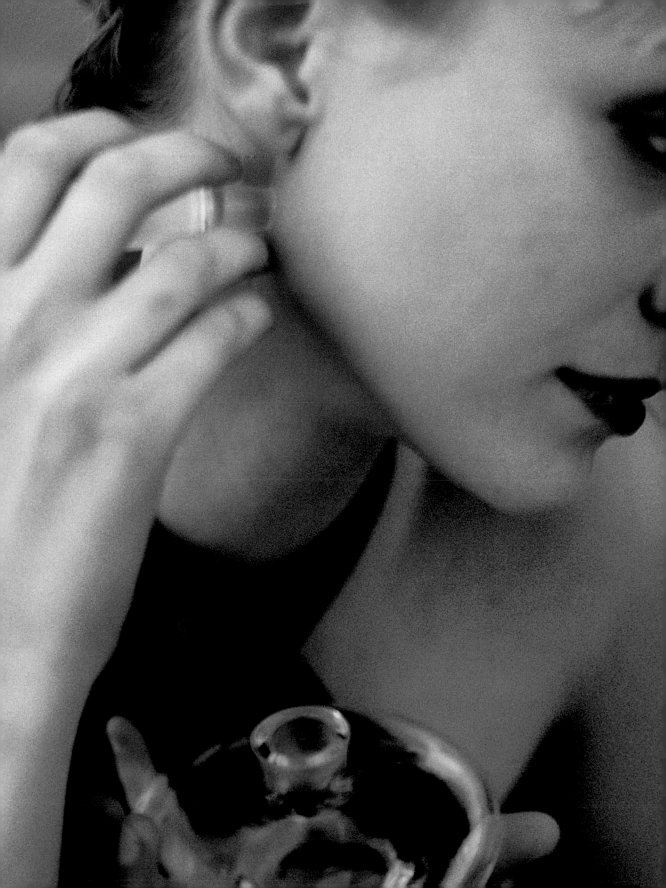

- **Be aware that your body gives out different scents at different times**—totally without your permission. There's bucketloads of evidence to suggest women smell differently when ovulating (i.e., at their most fertile). Your average man tends to agree, if not consciously. Lots of experiments prove men find women far more attractive and attainable when ovulating than at other times of the month.
- **Sit with your legs open** It works for both senses, if for wildly different reasons. Here, I'm suggesting guys do it because it takes advantage of the way pheromones are released. The male pheromone is called androsterone—its well-known cousin is testosterone. Androsterone is released from the armpits and groin, and it's one reason why sexually aggressive men tend to sit with their arms behind their head, legs planted firmly apart, and body facing toward the

Try **telling a sexy story** and see if your dinner date starts to **chew faster** and take **bigger mouthfuls** of food.

woman they admire. You might not be sure why you're doing it, but you've seen it done in movies and besides, it seems to work. Absolutely right, it does! It's a remarkably effective pose because it allows the pheromones released from Scent Central—your groin and armpit—to waft forward and work their magic.

- **Wear your own perfume** Your body has produced its own unique designer scent. It's free and readily accessible. Simply lean forward, insert a finger into your vagina and dab the secretions wherever you'd normally dab perfume. Female pheromones, called capulins, are released in our presweat glands and vaginal secretions. Yes, it takes courage, but do it once and you'll never go back. Besides, the only equally effective pheromone-based alternative is to rub your hand under an armpit and wipe that over your face or neck. I can't speak for you, but, quite frankly, I'd rather do the former.

THE TASTE OF SEX

Five thousand years ago, a woman sat in the prehistoric equivalent of a bathroom and applied pigment to color her lips—the first example of the true reason behind a lot of beauty rituals: to mimic the sexual organs in a bid to arouse a potential partner. Reddening our lips sends a distinct nonverbal signal of sexual arousal (the inner labia become bright red just prior to orgasm). To make an even clearer association, we also ensure they're slick, wet, and glossy, mirroring the increased lubrication of the female genitals which occurs when aroused. True, you probably won't find colors called "Luscious Labia" or "Va--va-voom Vagina" at the lipstick counter, but check out the lips featured in any high-profile lip-gloss/stick ad campaign, and it doesn't take too much imagination to see the model's mouth resembles a vagina turned the other way round!

Minus make-up, both sexes lick their lips when presented with someone or something they find arousing. Lots of women do it deliberately, with dramatic effect (though don't overplay it unless you want to look like you're a refugee from a girlie mag).

What happens when you meet someone you're attracted to?

The body moves into "plump" mode: the blood flows faster, plumping up the right parts to make them look fuller and more attractive. Just as the genitals engorge with blood and deepen in color when aroused, so do our lips turn red and become bigger. This (handily) increases their sensitivity, making us nicely primed for a possible kissing session. Try telling a sexy story and see if your dinner date starts to chew faster and take bigger mouthfuls of food. If they do, they're not just wolfing it down to hurry up the part where they get to take you home, but their lips have also become supersensitive to stimulation so that all touch feels good. We subconsciously invent all kinds of socially acceptable ways to touch our own mouth and lips when aroused. An obvious way to turn someone on using our mouths: eat food suggestively. Eating with our fingers and then licking them afterward advertises our talents for what might be in store later.

Make it work for you…

- **Let nature do its stuff** Don't disguise the natural messages your bodies are trying to send each other by smoking, eating strong food, drinking strong-scented alcohol, or using breath fresheners. Just as smell is a great dictator of who should or shouldn't get together, so are your breath and saliva important biological messengers.

- **Trust your first kiss** Plenty of people use the first kiss as a technical litmus test: if the kiss is good, the sex will be as well. Others use it to test for chemistry: if sparks don't fly, perhaps it's just friendship. Both have evidence to back them up. Pucker up to kiss someone you're attracted to and sebaceous glands in your mouth and the corners of your lips release semiochemicals, which are designed to stimulate sexual excitement. These combine with your own unique saliva "fingerprint," and the end result is passed on during kissing. It's a bit like swapping business cards listing your personal credentials, except a hell of a lot sexier! Most people know if they're going to be suited physically after their first full kiss. The way we kiss someone for the first time also has a direct effect on whether a relationship progresses further.

- **Make it memorable** Start by kissing with your mouths closed, keeping the pressure soft and gentle. Make the kisses a little harder, then part your lips slightly to let the chemicals communicate. How warm are their breath, lips, and tongue? If they're aroused, everything should feel nicely heated up. If instead everything's cool or cold, you might be turned on but they're definitely not.

- **Read their lips** Most people kiss the way they like to be kissed. Be passive for moments at a time and let them take the lead. It's then simply a matter of imitating their technique. Be aware of how hard or soft they're kissing you, how fast, and what they're (ahem) suggesting with their tongue. If their technique's awful and you'd rather they follow you, pull back for a second, look them in the eye, and say, "Let me kiss you. I've been waiting forever for this so let me have my way for a minute". Then lean in, take over, and hope they get the hint and follow your lead.

Sleeping together

Though it's entirely possible to fake feelings while awake, you can't fake anything when you're asleep. This is why some experts believe the way you sleep together can reveal lots about your true emotions and the state of your relationship. It makes sense when you think about it: the closer you are, the closer you're likely to sleep; if you fear someone's about to leave, chances are you'll cling on tight; if you're the one thinking of leaving, you'll create distance between you. The positions below are loosely based on research by California psychiatrist Mark Goulston. As he admits, they're not accurate relationship indicators, but they can give clues.

LOVING SPOON (top left)
The classic "happily married" position: loving but still wanting to be physically close. One of you lies on your side, the other snuggles up behind, pulling you close by draping an arm around your waist. Few couples hug or spoon during sleep if they're sexually frustrated or resentful. (The partner who's not eager for sex is worried any sign of affection will be interpreted as an invitation; the other gets the message any touch is unwelcome so stops trying.)

HONEYMOON (top right)
Ridiculously romantic (though lots would add claustrophobic), this is the pose of new lovers smack bang in the honeymoon part of their relationship (the I-can't-believe-I've-found-you bit). The full-length whole body hug—facing each other, every part touching—sends three signals: a desire to connect on all levels, a need for reassurance (by hanging on possessively, they can't run away), and total commitment to each other and the relationship. Yes, it might all end in tears, but right now you're dreaming of white picket fences and 2.2 children.

BUTT TO BUTT (bottom left)
Studies prove it's far more comfortable to sleep solo, yet few dispute the joy of sleeping with someone you love. This is a good compromise. You're lying on your own side of the bed with plenty of room to move, but your butts touch. Couples who sleep like this are in good shape: it's pretty impressive that you're maintaining contact with each other even when unconscious and back to back! Awake, you're likely to be affectionate and not afraid of intimacy.

DANGEROUS DISTANCE (bottom right)
You're at opposite sides of the bed, back to back. One or both of your arms cross over your body, forming a partial arm block. Not only are you protecting yourself emotionally by literally covering your heart, but you're also reducing the chance of accidentally touching each other while asleep. This is the "post argument" position. If you're sleeping like this permanently, watch out. Lots of space between you as you sleep usually translates to emotional distance during waking hours.

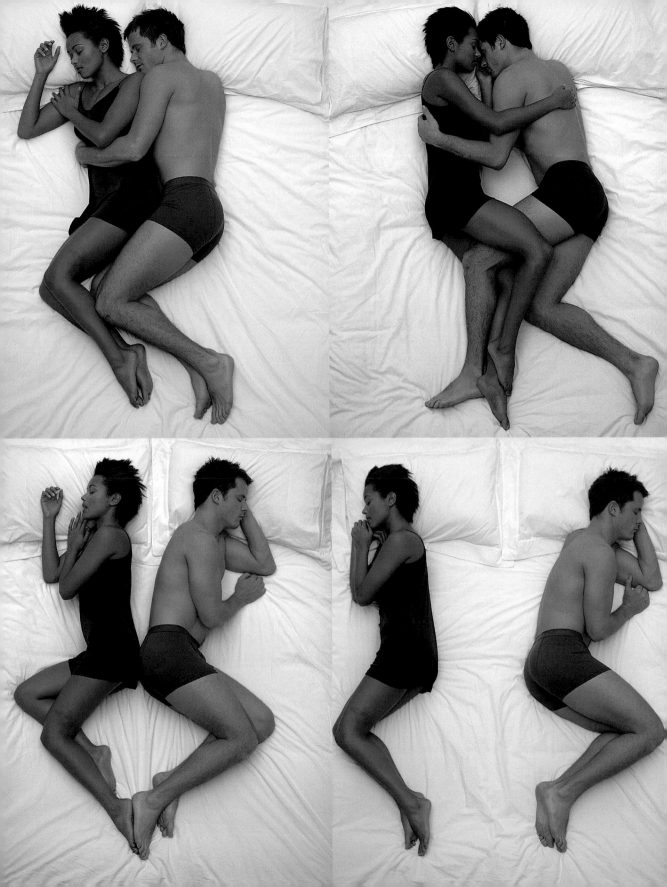

What to say the very next day...

Many a great relationship has been halted in full stride by a miserable morning after. Act too eager and you risk being branded as desperate; play it too cool and you risk losing them. The solution? Keep it light and friendly. To make sense of the morning-after madness, here's some solutions to the most frequently asked questions.

I've woken up to find her looking gorgeous, if slightly disheveled and hungover, in my bed. Every part of me—one in particular—wants to wake her up and do it all over again, but I'm scared she'll think all I want her for is sex. Are we supposed to have breakfast first?

Dive straight in before she's woken up and you'll set the mood for the morning: sexy. That's (obviously) not a bad thing, but if you do really like her just make sure it's more soppy-sexy than lusty-sexy because she's likely to be feeling a little vulnerable. Everyone who's got an emotional investment in a relationship feels delicate the day after you've just done it. You're teenagers again, wondering if they still like you, worrying if you were good enough/too good (aka slutty)/thin/hard/tight enough. Thankfully, there's an instant solution to dissolving all those fears: spoon her. No one spoons comfortably the morning after if they're not interested in at least giving the relationship a try. What? You have no idea what I'm talking about? Spooning's easy. Lie on your side facing her back and simply snuggle into each other like spoons (see p.183, top left). Connected but facing in the same direction, you don't have to make eye contact (or smell each other's breath) so can wake up, get used to each other, and have conversations without ever having to meet anyone's eye. Once you've been sufficiently smoochy, that's the time to make your move sexually. Start by running your hands over her body appreciatively—her arms, the curve of her thighs, her tummy—and see how she responds. If she arches toward your touch like a cat, you're fine to move on to touching the good parts. Ditto, if she turns around to ravage you. If, however, she brushes your hands away or you feel her body tense with nerves or disapproval, she needs bucketloads of reassurance as well as coffee. Give up, get up, and put the coffee on.

They're leaving early and going straight to work. Where should I say goodbye so I look interested but not desperate? Is it better to stay in bed or get up and see them to the door? P.S. I'm not very good at prancing around naked.

It depends on the mood, so play it by ear. If they're getting ready in the bedroom and talking to you, it makes sense to stay in bed. It also makes sense to stay put if they don't seem eager. But if they've been especially huggy and/or sexy and there's been plenty of "If you knew how hard it is to leave you..." stuff, kiss them goodbye from under the covers, then just as they hit the front door, shout out, "Hold on a minute!". Grab something which barely covers (like a t-shirt) and hold it in front of you as you pad after them in your bare feet. Deliver one final devastatingly sexy kiss with your (sort of) naked body pressed firmly against their fully clothed one, then smile wickedly, stand behind the door, and open it for them to exit. If this doesn't make them come back for more, nothing will.

And while we're on the topic, what if…

- **She seems loving but didn't seem turned on or to enjoy it** It could be nerves. It could be that she takes time to get used to your technique—most women take at least 3–4 sessions before they'll relax enough to orgasm. Or it could be she's plucking up the courage to tell you what she really needs to make it happen. If her previous lover knew she liked anal stimulation during oral sex and her body got used to it, it's become an orgasm trigger for her. She's so used to climaxing that way, she finds it hard to push herself over the edge without it. She might not feel comfortable enough to confess her "trigger" immediately, for fear you might judge her. Speed up the process by making it as comfortable as possible for the two of you to talk about your needs and desires.

- **He asked if I had an orgasm and I lied and said yes** What he was really asking was: Do you think I'm a good lover? Which means you could have answered by saying something like, "Ummmmmm—that was just delicious! I l-o-v-e-d it. I know I didn't have an orgasm, but it takes me a little while to get used to someone new. Mind you, you're so good at it, it'll be no time at all!" Easy! Shame that instead, you found yourself mumbling "Huh? Oh, mmmm" as you hid your face in his chest. Bad girl! Continue and you've sown the seed for a nice little pattern of dishonesty. Fix it by being honest next time. Say, "That was fabulous. I could feel myself hovering but couldn't quite get there." Unless he's a complete twit, his next question will be, "What do I do next time to get it right?". At which point you…tell him. If you're thinking, I can't say any of that because I wasn't even close to climax, don't panic. You're better off building sexual confidence and opening the lines of communication than perfecting technique.

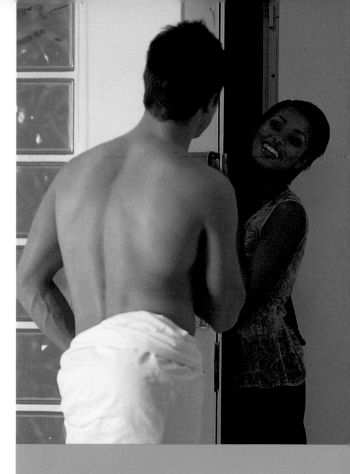

Deliver one final **devastatingly sexy kiss** with your (sort of) **naked body pressed** firmly against their fully-clothed one, then **smile wickedly.**

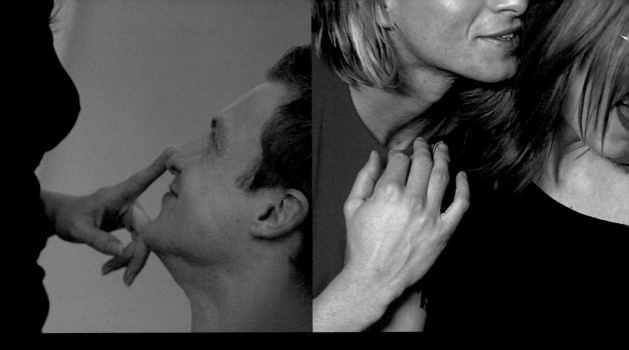

Touch me there

A touch can magnify a message three times over. Whether we want to convey affection (top left), ownership, and protection (top right), or sexual possessiveness (bottom right), our fingertips do the job without us ever having to open our mouths. Touch can also be used to self-comfort (main picture), or to show that we mean business (bottom left).

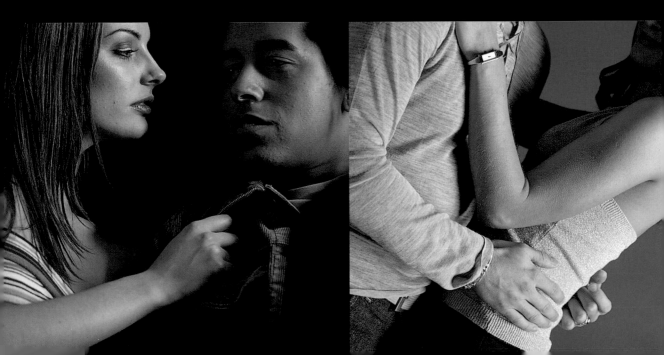

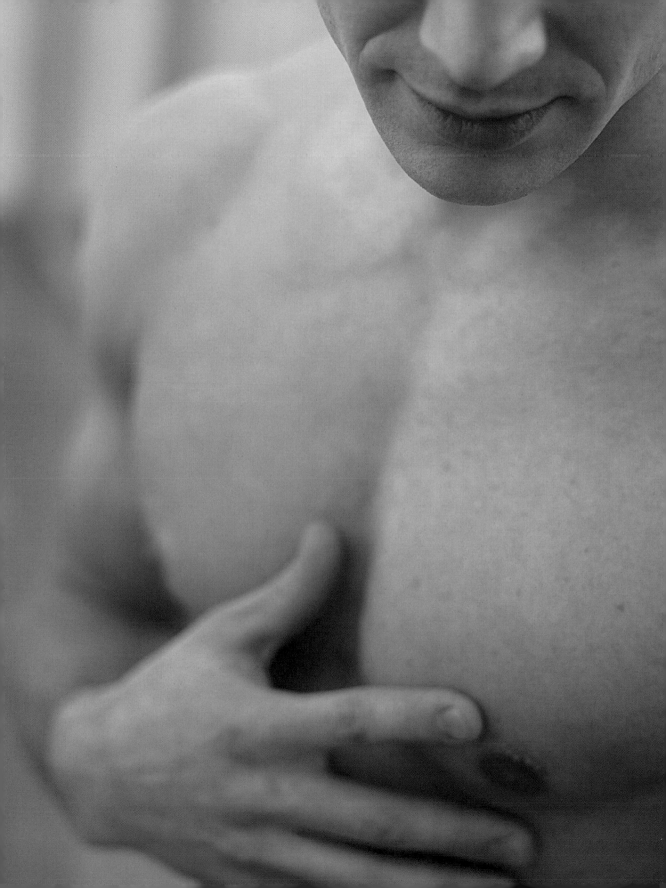

Index

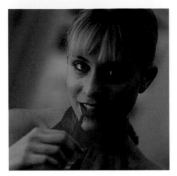

Acknowledgments

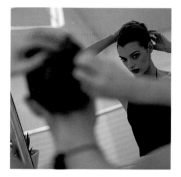

The author would like to thank the following people:

First and foremost, thanks to my publisher, DK, who has, as always, treated me like a princess. Thanks go to Corinne Roberts for unwavering and constant support and encouragement, along with highly motivational (rather liquid) lunches; ditto, my lovely friend Deborah Wright; Christopher Davis, for having faith in my projects; Serena Stent and Rachel Kempster, for letting the world know about them; and Emma Forge and Carole Ash, for doing everything in their power to make the book look great. Enormous thanks especially to my long-suffering editor, Peter Jones, who bolstered me up or calmed me down, depending on what was needed, and who never once complained while I made myriad pointless, miniscule changes that absolutely no one else would notice but me.

Nigel and Bev, from XAB, for once again working their magic to make the book look sensational; and Janeanne Gilchrist for the innovative photography.

Vicki McIvor, my much-loved and hardworking agent, whose 24/7 professional and emotional support is appreciated far more than she will ever know.

My family, who is in my thoughts every second of the day and who I carry with me in my heart wherever I go.

My friends who, once again, not only shared their personal anecdotes, read copy, and road-tested techniques, but who also generously forgave me for, yet again, being unavailable for fun and frolics. Where's the party guys?

DK would like to thank Laurence Errington for the index and Constance Novis for proofreading.

A lot of people stop flirting once they're in a relationship. **Don't.** The couple **that plays** together **stays together**.

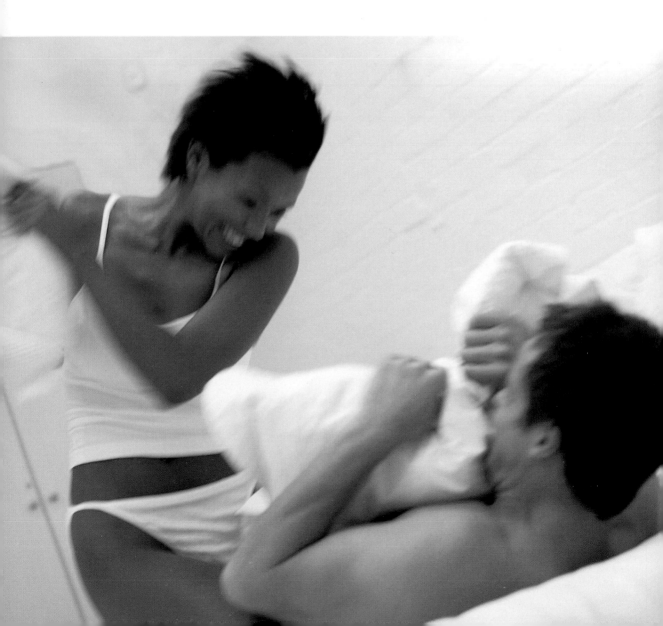